Recipes Mediterranean inspired

Lina Khatib

Interior designer/ health conscience

Recipes Mediterranean Inspired

ISBN
Paperback: 978-1-967668-52-6
Hardcover: 978-1-967668-53-3

The book will be dedicated to love
♡ as these recipes were inspired by
a love state, in a loving home.

You are what you eat!

Cooking requires motivation to be healthy. Dedicate some time to it. Preparing meal at home is priceless. After tasting many dishes around the world, I concluded that simplicity and freshness are the best way to live a healthier and happier life.

My dishes are Westernized, inspired by Mediterranean cuisine and based on those repeated ingredients: beans, grains, oil, lemon, garlic, onions, etc.

Science has proven that eating less is good for your health. Therefore, fasting and intermittent fasting are beneficial for the whole being on many levels. The body will be in a reset mode and will function better.

This booklet is for people who commit to eating less and healthier. Even though carbs are good for the hormone serotonin, we can still have carbs by substituting starchy foods like bread and rice with grains and legumes or by simply balancing the entire diet by eating everything in moderation.

Let's toss bad snacks like potato chips and others, have more walnuts, dates, dried figs, popcorn, or mixed nuts as snacks, and introduce more beans or legumes into our diet.

Let's start to be healthy!

Enjoy!

Ingredients in these recipes are intended for 2 people. You can multiply the amount for the extra count. This booklet is not meant for beginner cooks.

All recipes use the white onion, unless otherwise mentioned.

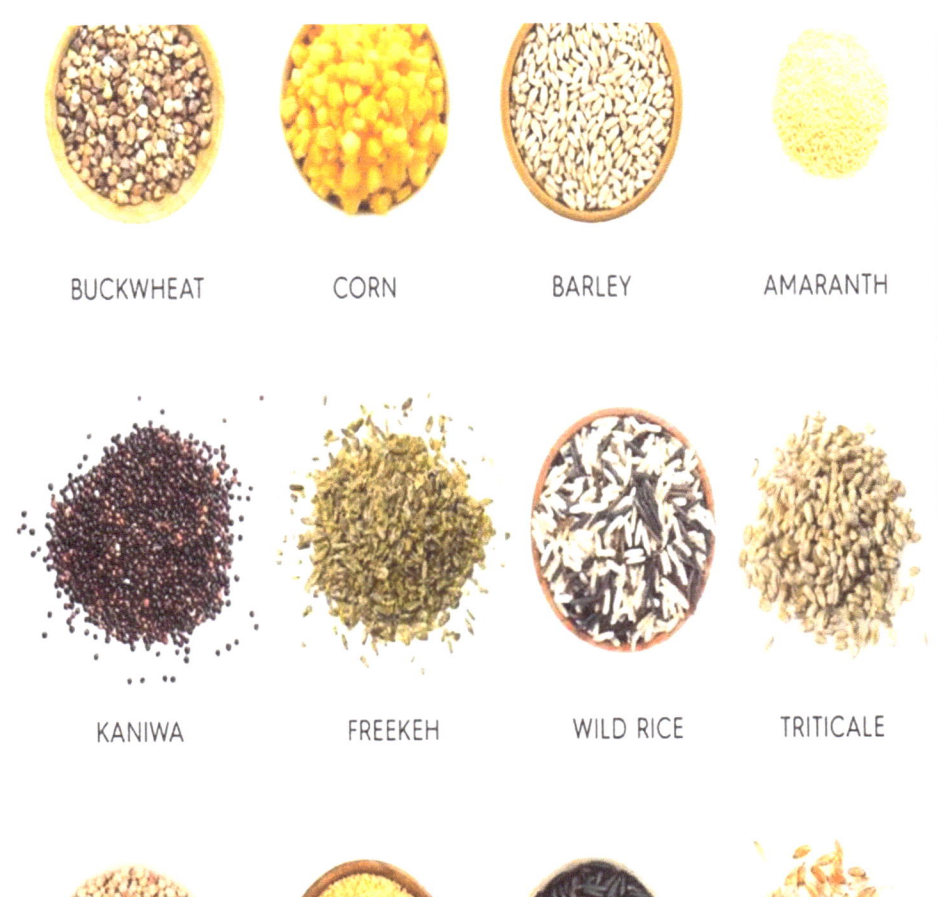

BUCKWHEAT   CORN   BARLEY   AMARANTH

KANIWA   FREEKEH   WILD RICE   TRITICALE

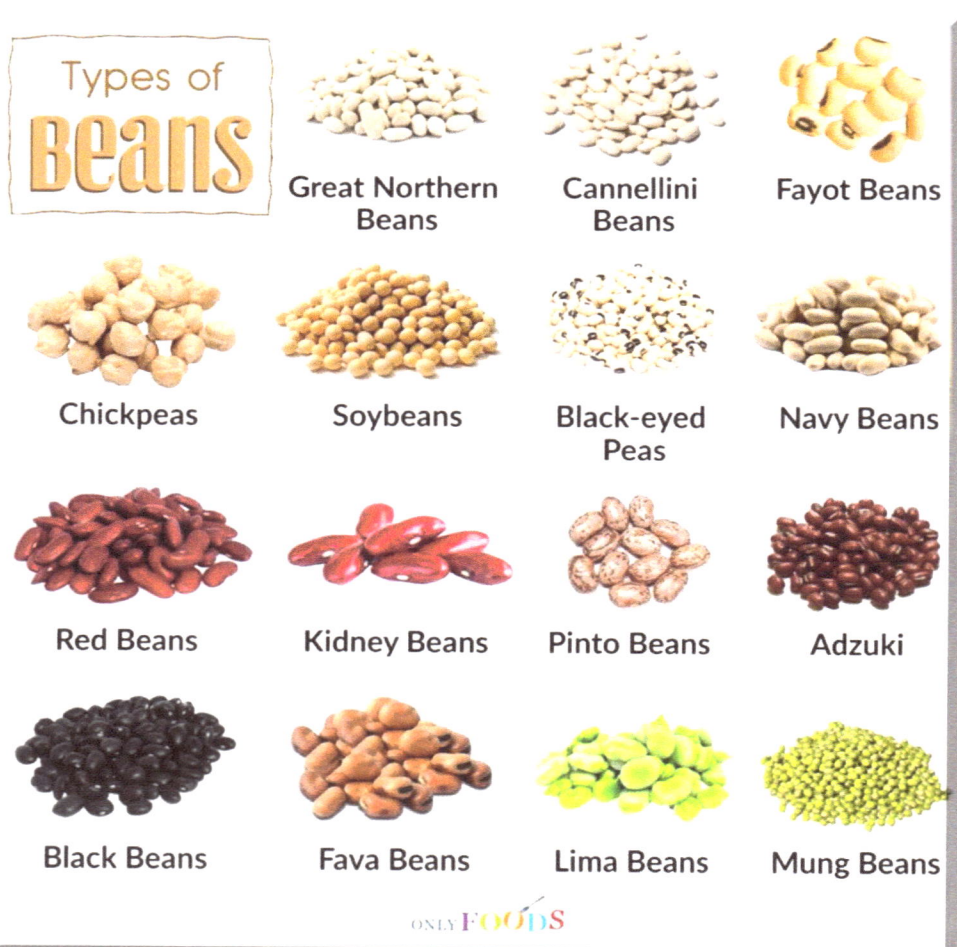

Types of **Beans**

Great Northern Beans

Cannellini Beans

Fayot Beans

Chickpeas

Soybeans

Black-eyed Peas

Navy Beans

Red Beans

Kidney Beans

Pinto Beans

Adzuki

Black Beans

Fava Beans

Lima Beans

Mung Beans

ONLY FOODS

As a health-conscious individual, I have lived all my life looking for a better way to have food in me, as I do believe that you are what you eat. Food has a huge positive impact on your health if chosen correctly . I have cooked many recipes from books written by chefs all around the globe. I concluded that meals made with fresh ingredients, including plenty of beans **and** grains, are the best. I was inspired by a lot of existing recipes and made my own. The way I see them is the best. Basically, these recipes are my version of old recipes, but they are done fresh and in a new way. My version! Here is why beans are important to your health. Beans contain amino acids, which are the protein building blocks that the body uses to heal and to make new tissues, such as bones, muscles, hair, skin, and blood.

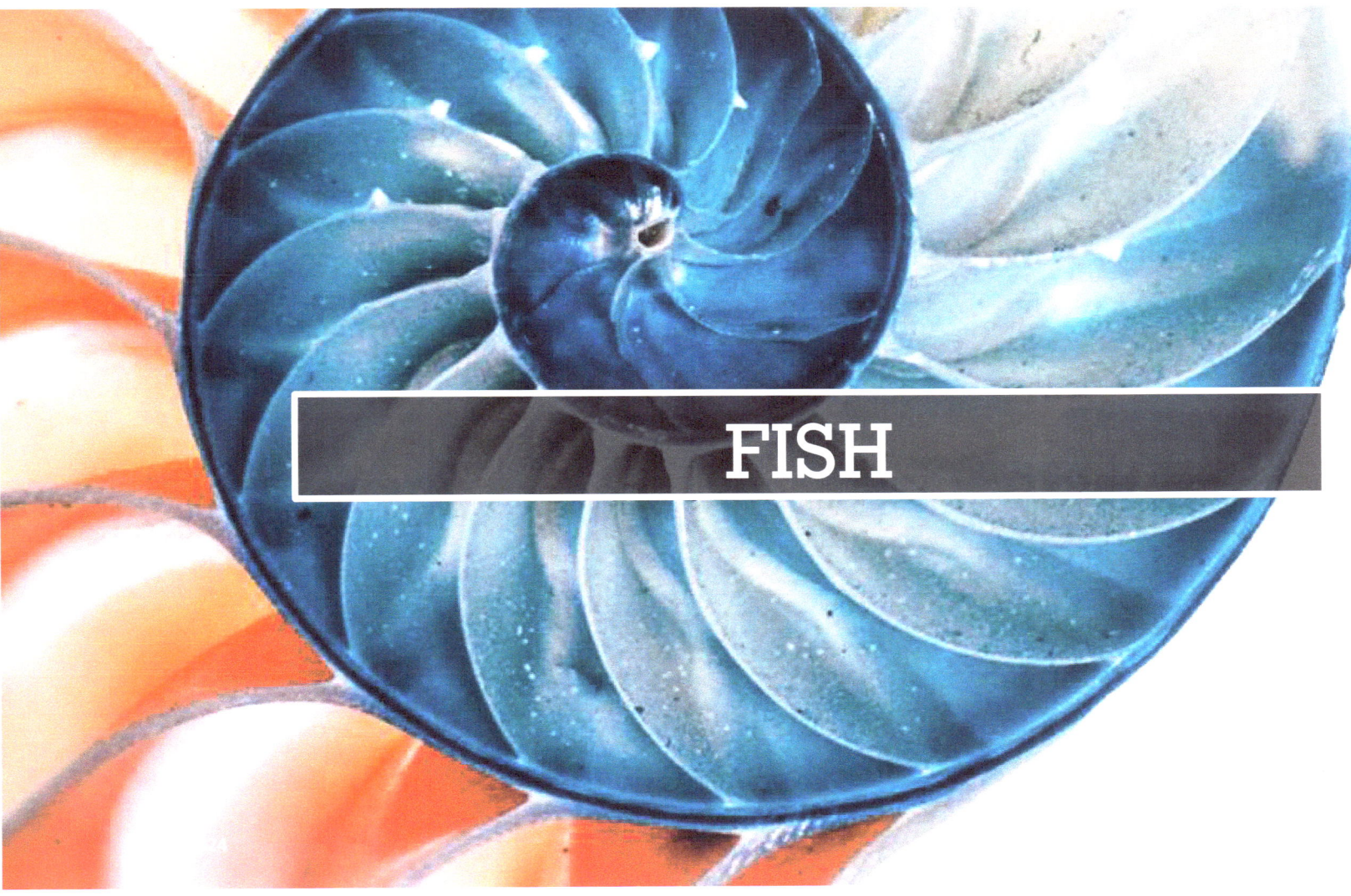

FISH

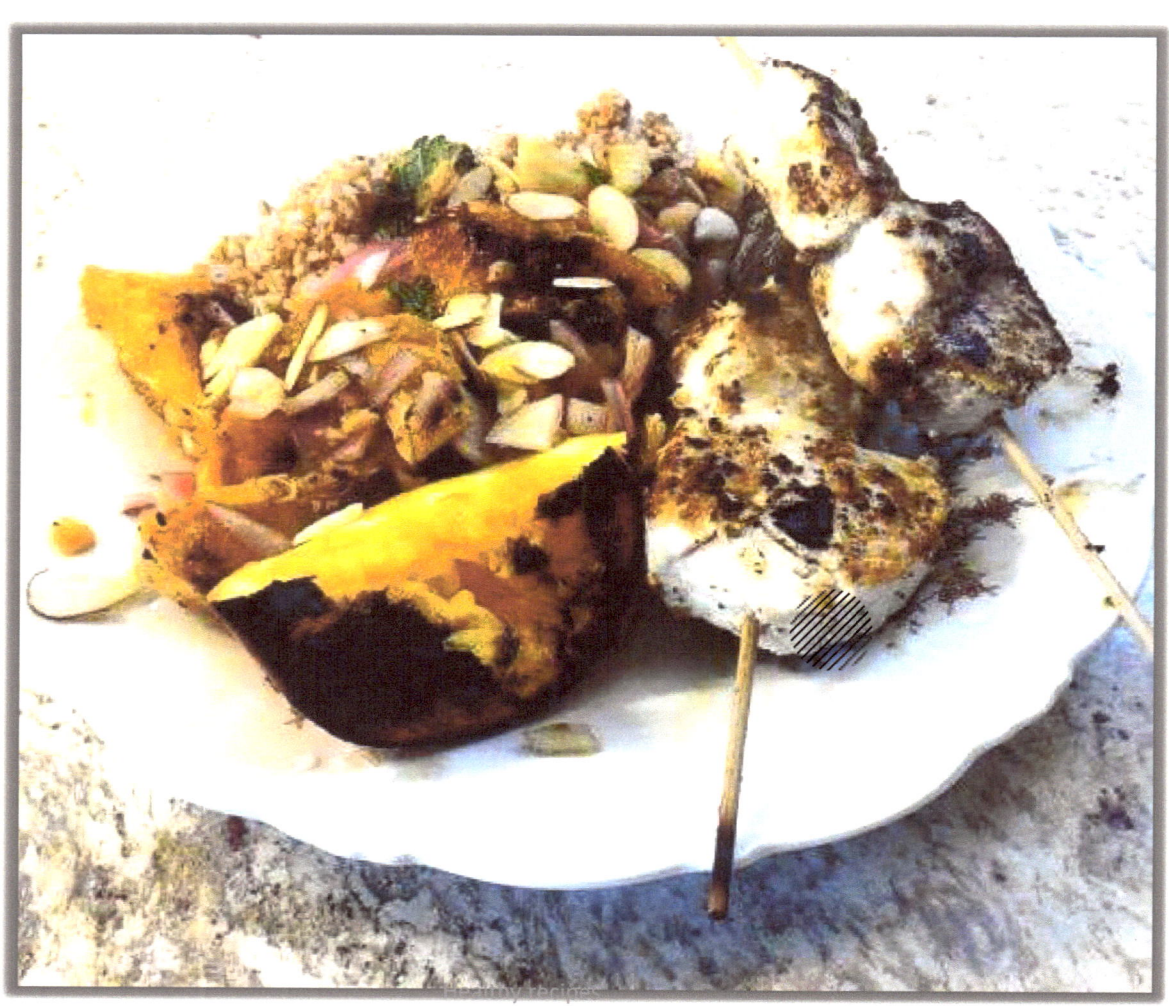

1. TUNA. BARLEY.ALMONDS.

Ingredients:
Sprinkle with salt and pepper 1 Pound of Tuna fish cut into cubes, marinated with ¼ cup of vinegar, 1 TBSP of mustard and ¼ cup of olive oil for at least 1 hour. Skewer the tuna and Grill for 18 minutes.
1 cup of barley boiled and strained.
1 TBSP of mustard.
2 TBSP of olive oil.
1 TBSP of sliced almonds.
A squeeze of 1 lemon.
1/4 cup of vinegar.
Salt and black pepper.
Mix all ingredients in a bowl, add the salt and pepper then squeeze 1 lemon.
Serve the mix alongside the grilled tuna.

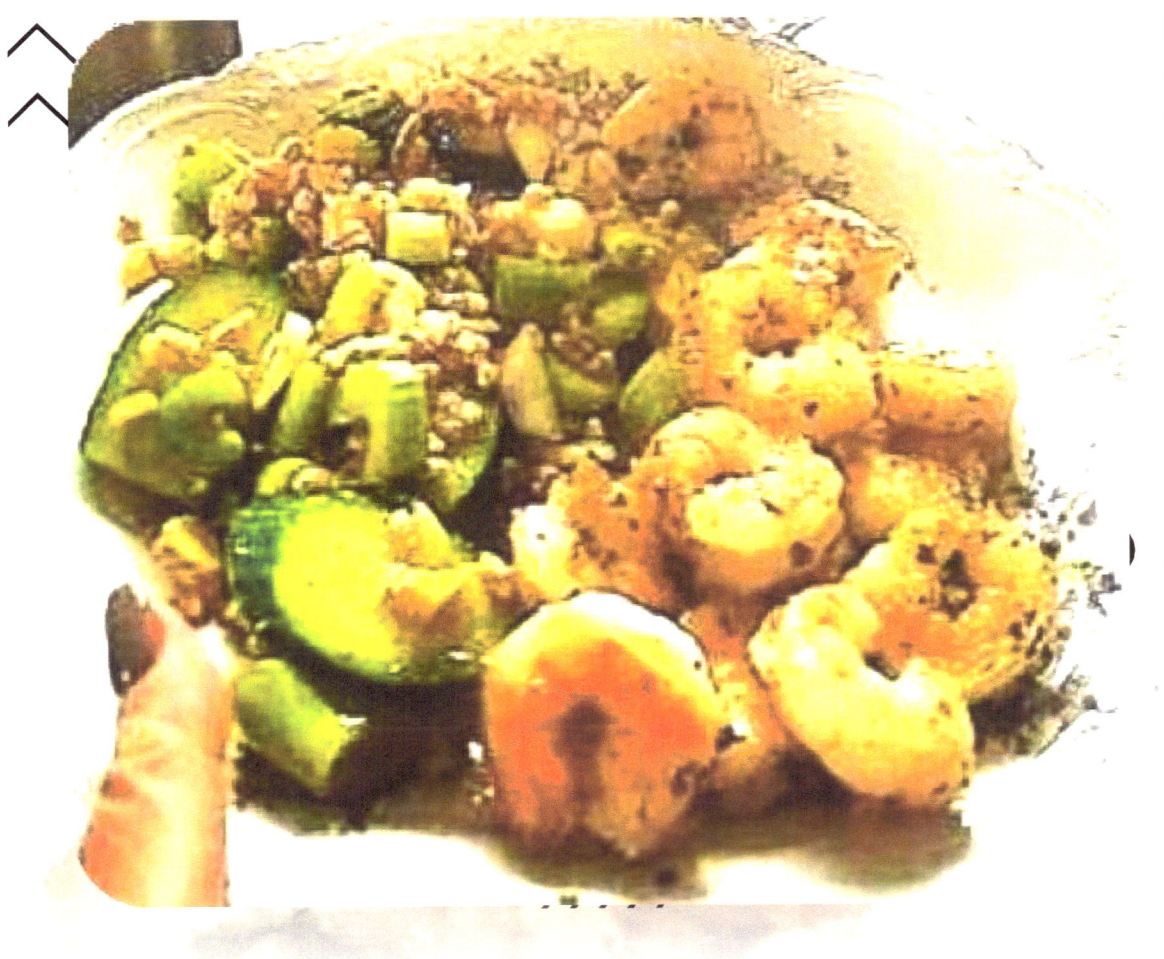

2. SHRIMP. BARLEY. CUCUMBER

Ingredients:
1 pound or half a kilo of precooked shrimp brushed with 2 TBSP of sesame oil, 2 tablespoons of rice vinegar, salt, and pepper, grilled on medium heat for 4 minutes on each side . Set aside.
1 cucumber, sliced into rounds.
6 stems of chopped green onions.
3 stalk of celery.
2 TBSP of rice vinegar.
2 cloves of garlic.
¾ cup of barley boiled and strained.
1 TBSP cf sesame oil.
1 TSP of sesame seeds
Combine all ingredients in a bowl and add a pinch of salt and pepper.
Serve alongside the shrimp.

Recipes Mediterranean Inspired

3. TUNA. OKRA. BEANS

Ingredients:
Grill 1 pound of tuna cut lengthwise, brushed with olive oil, salt, and pepper for 9 minutes a side or until the desired doneness.
8 large okra sliced in half, brushed with olive oil, salt, and pepper, and grilled on medium heat until they are soft and done.
½ cup boiled kidney beans, strained.
1 TBSP of Kalamata olives.
2 TBSP of olive oil.
½ a white onion, diced small.
1 TBSP of granulated mustard.
2 cloves of chopped garlic.
Combine all ingredients in a bowl. Add a final touch of salt and pepper.
Serve alongside the grilled tuna.

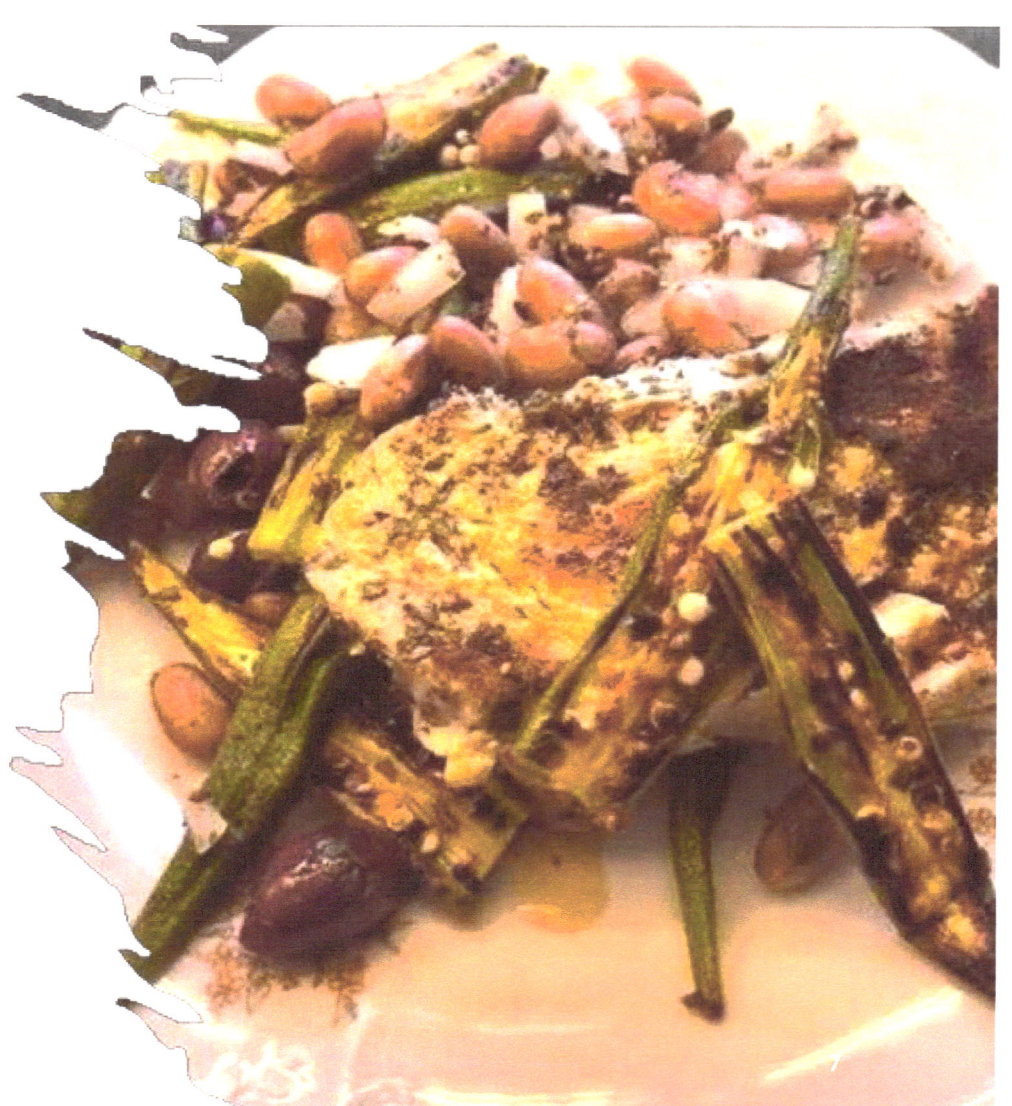

4. COD. SWEET POTATO. CORN. PICKLES.

Ingredients:
1 pound or ½ kilo of cod or any white flaky fish, brushed with olive oil, salt and pepper. Grilled for 17 minutes, to be flipped only once.
½ a cup of frozen corn thawed.
A few leaves of fresh basil.
5 cornichon pickles sliced into rounds.
½ a white onion, chopped small.
2 sweet potatoes sliced in half, brushed with olive oil, salt and pepper. Grilled on medium heat for an hour.
1 TBSP of balsamic vinegar.
2 TBSP of olive oil.
Combine and mix all ingredients In a bowl, add the final touch of salt and pepper.
 Serve alongside the grilled fish.

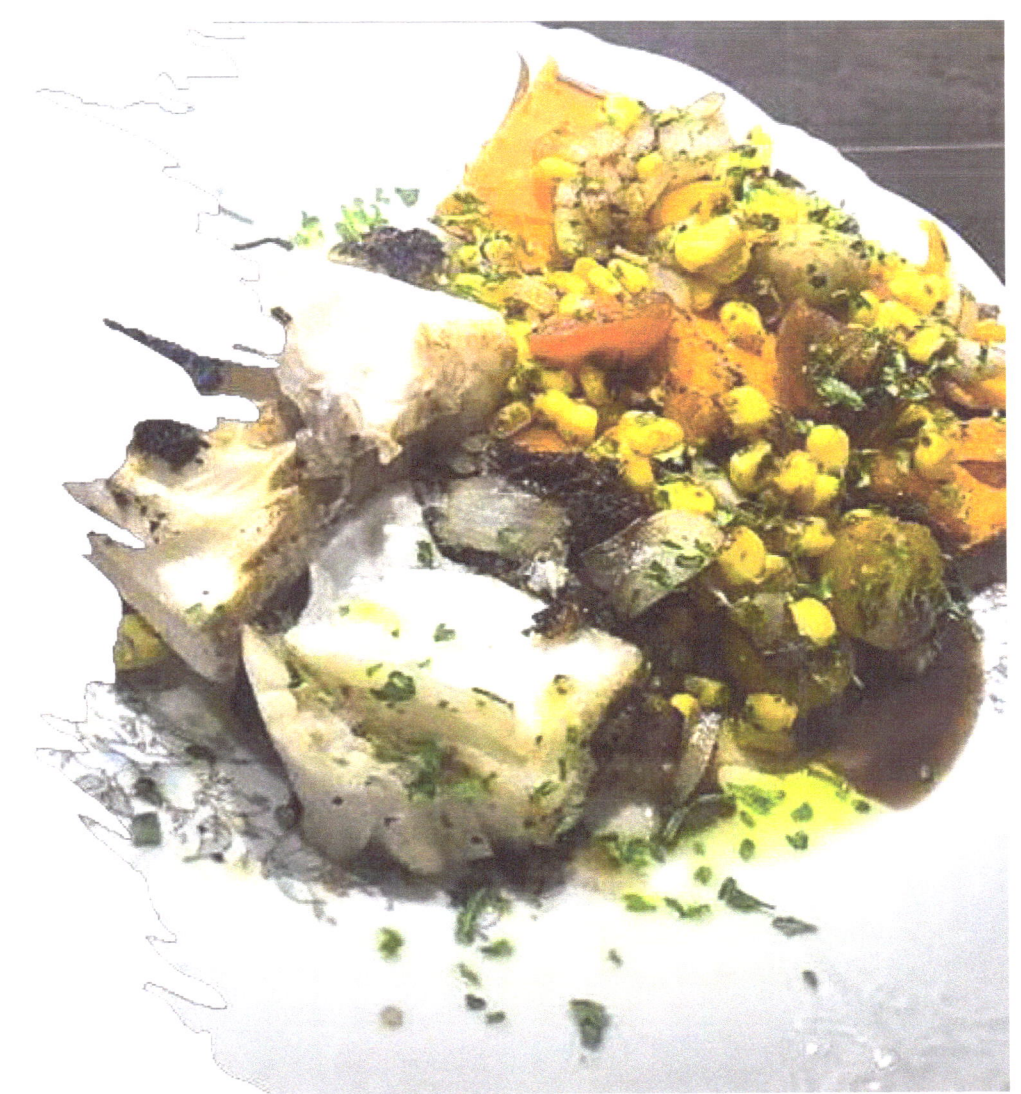

5. TUNA SKEWERS. CAPERS. CORN. BROCCOLI

Ingredients:

1 pound or ½ kilo of dense fish or tuna cut into cubes, marinated for at least 1 hour with ¼ cup of white vinegar and ¼ cup of olive oil with a pinch of salt and black pepper and 4 cloves of minced garlic.

Put the cubed marinated tuna on skewers with the quarters of one onion and the cut green peppers.

½ a cup of frozen corn

½ a white onion diced into small pieces.

3 tablespoons of olive oil and 1 tablespoon of capers.

2 stems of grilled broccoli brushed with olive oil, salt and pepper.

1 lemon squeezed for juice

4 cloves of garlic, minced.

Mix all ingredients in a bowl, add a pinch of salt and black pepper.

Serve all alongside grilled onions, tuna and pepper skewers and you can.

Serve alongside grilled broccoli.

Recipes Mediterranean Inspired

6. COD. BULGUR

Ingredients:

Grilled cod or any Mediterranean flaky white fish for 17 minutes after brushing it with a little olive oil, salt, or pepper.

¾ cup of bulgur or cracked wheat boiled until done, strained.

¼ cup of pitted, diced olives. Either green or black olives work.

¼ TSP of harissa paste

Diced ½ white onion

Salt and pepper.

Olive oil

A sprinkle of dried oregano.

Dried tomatoes cut into 4 pieces.

Combine bulgur, harissa, onion, oil, and olives in a bowl.

Line a small ramekin with Saran Wrap, Add a big serving spoon of the mix into this ramekin, flip so you will have a domed shape or half a ball. Serve alongside the grilled fish.

Sprinkle all with dried oregano. Decorate with dried tomatoes on top.

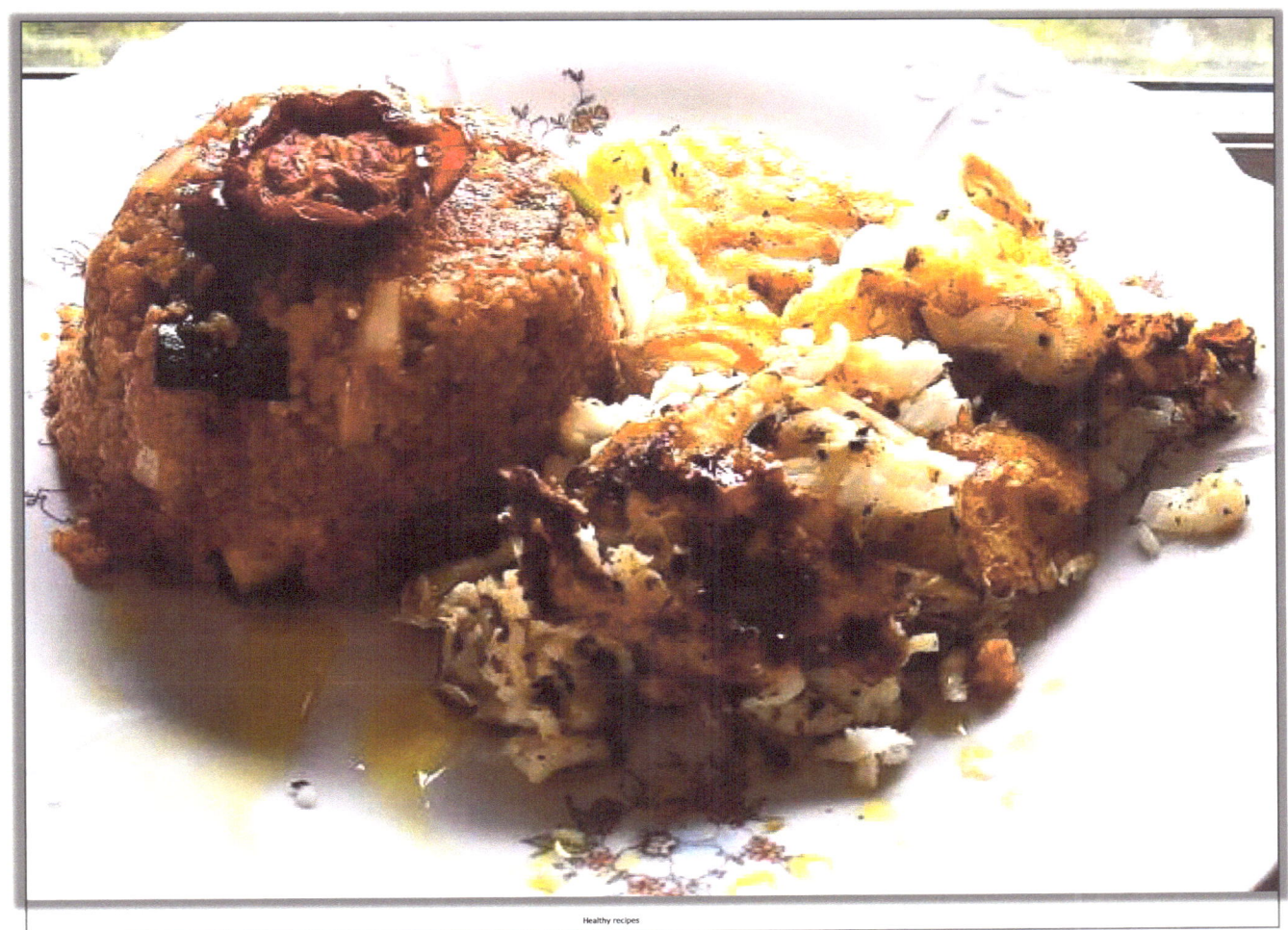

Healthy recipes

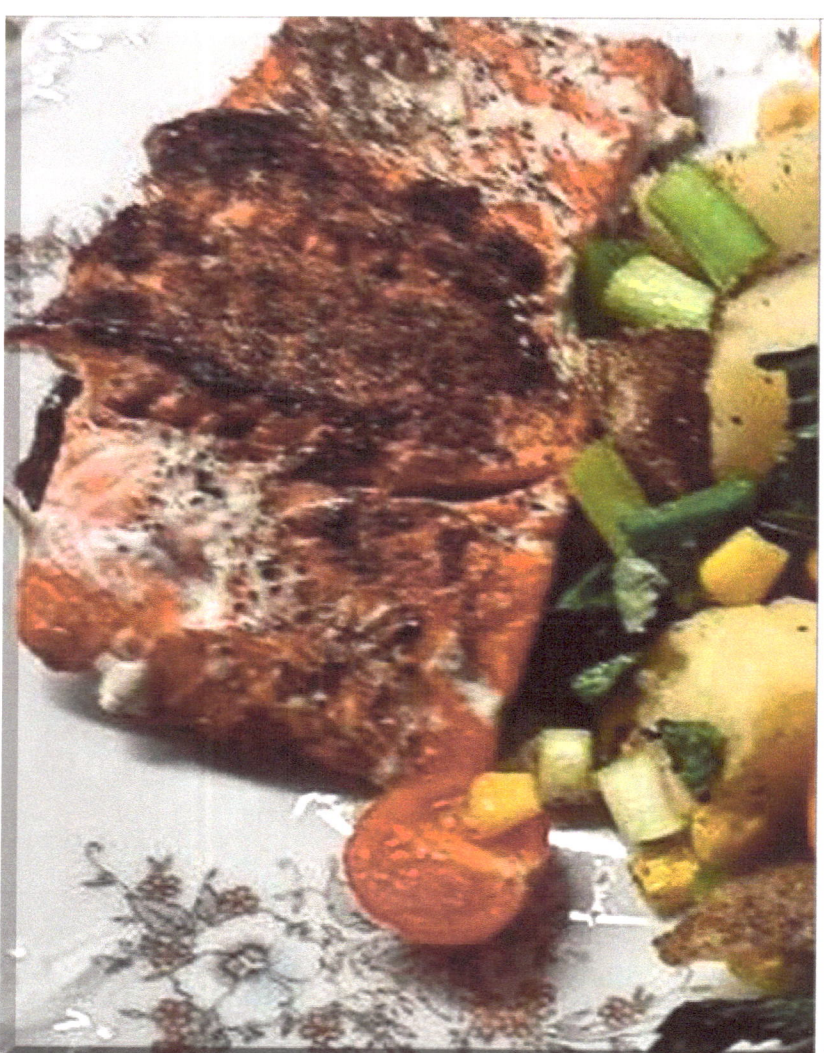

7. SALMON POTATO. VEGGIES

Ingredients:
1 pound or ½ kilo of salmon, brushed with olive oil, salt, and pepper. Grilled for 18 minutes, flip only once.
2 heads of mid-size potatoes boiled.
4 stems of green onions sliced into rounds
8 pieces of grape tomatoes or 1 head of regular-sized tomatoes, sliced into small pieces.
2 stems of collard greens or SILIK, diced into small pieces.
2 cloves of garlic, diced.
2 TBSP of olive oil
1 lemon squeezed for juice.
Combine and mix all ingredients, serve alongside the grilled salmon. Add a final touch of salt and pepper.

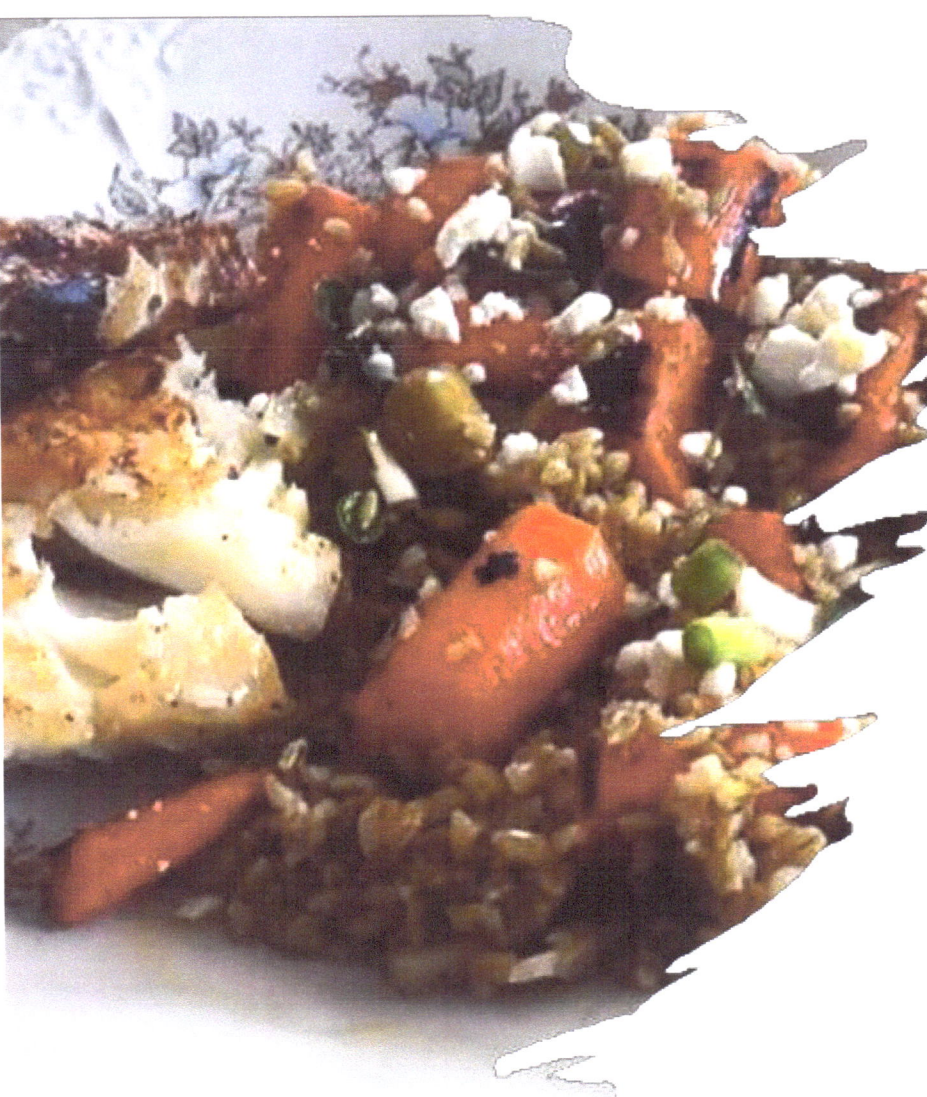

8. COD. WHEAT. CARROTS. OLIVES

Ingredients:
1 pound of cod or any flaky white fish, brushed with olive oil, salt, and pepper. Grilled for 17 minutes, flip only once.
3 carrots, brushed with olive oil, salt, and pepper. Cut into small chunks and grilled.
2 TBSP of green or Kalamata olives, pitted.
¾ cup of boiled whole wheat or barley.
¼ cup of feta cheese
4 stems of green onions, diced.
½ of a white onion, diced
2 TBSP balsamic vinegar
2 TBSP olive oil.
A few freshly chopped mint leaves.
Combine all ingredients and mix with balsamic and olive oil, and sprinkle with salt and pepper.
Serve alongside the grilled fish.

9. COD.
SWEET POTATO. BLACK BEANS.

Ingredients:

1 pound or ½ a kilo of cod or any white flaky fish, brushed with olive oil and sprinkled with salt and pepper. Grilled on medium heat for 17 minutes, flip only once.

¾ cup of pinto beans or black beans boiled and strained.

3 stems of diced green onions.

½ a bunch of diced cilantro.

2 tablespoons olive oil

1 lime juice

2 cloves of diced garlic

1 sweet potato, cut in half, brushed with olive oil, sprinkled with salt and pepper. Grilled for at least 50 minutes on medium heat.

Combine and mix all ingredients, sprinkle with salt and pepper, add lime juice and olive oil.

Serve alongside the grilled fish and potatoes.

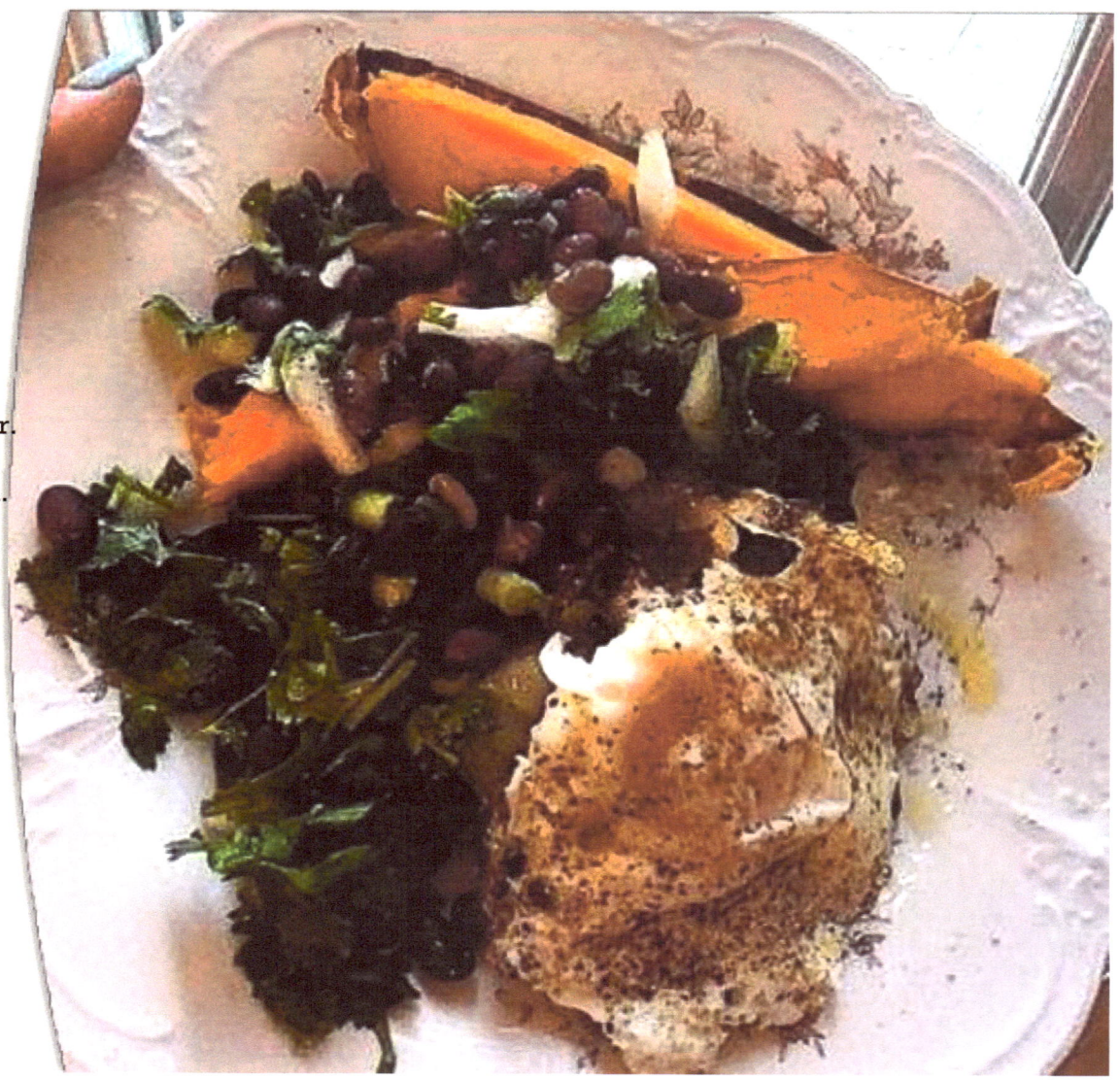

Recipes Mediterranean Inspired

10. COD. SPINACH. BARLEY

Ingredients:
1 pound or ½ a kilo of cod or any flaky white fish. Season with salt, pepper and sumac. Brush with olive oil then grill for 17 minutes on medium heat; turn only once.
¾ cup of barley, boiled, strained.
1 bunch of spinach or 1 bag of 1 pound of frozen spinach.
2 diced cloves of garlic
1 white onion, diced.
4 TBSP of olive oil.
4 TBSP of sumac.
¼ cup of white vinegar.
Zest of one lemon.
Sauté diced onions in a pan with 3 tablespoons of olive oil. When onions got wilt, add spinach, keep sautéing until spinach shrinks then add 3 TBSP of sumac, salt & pepper. When it's done, add the mixture to the barley in a bowl. Then, stir in ¼ cup of vinegar and the lemon zest.
Serve alongside the grilled fish.

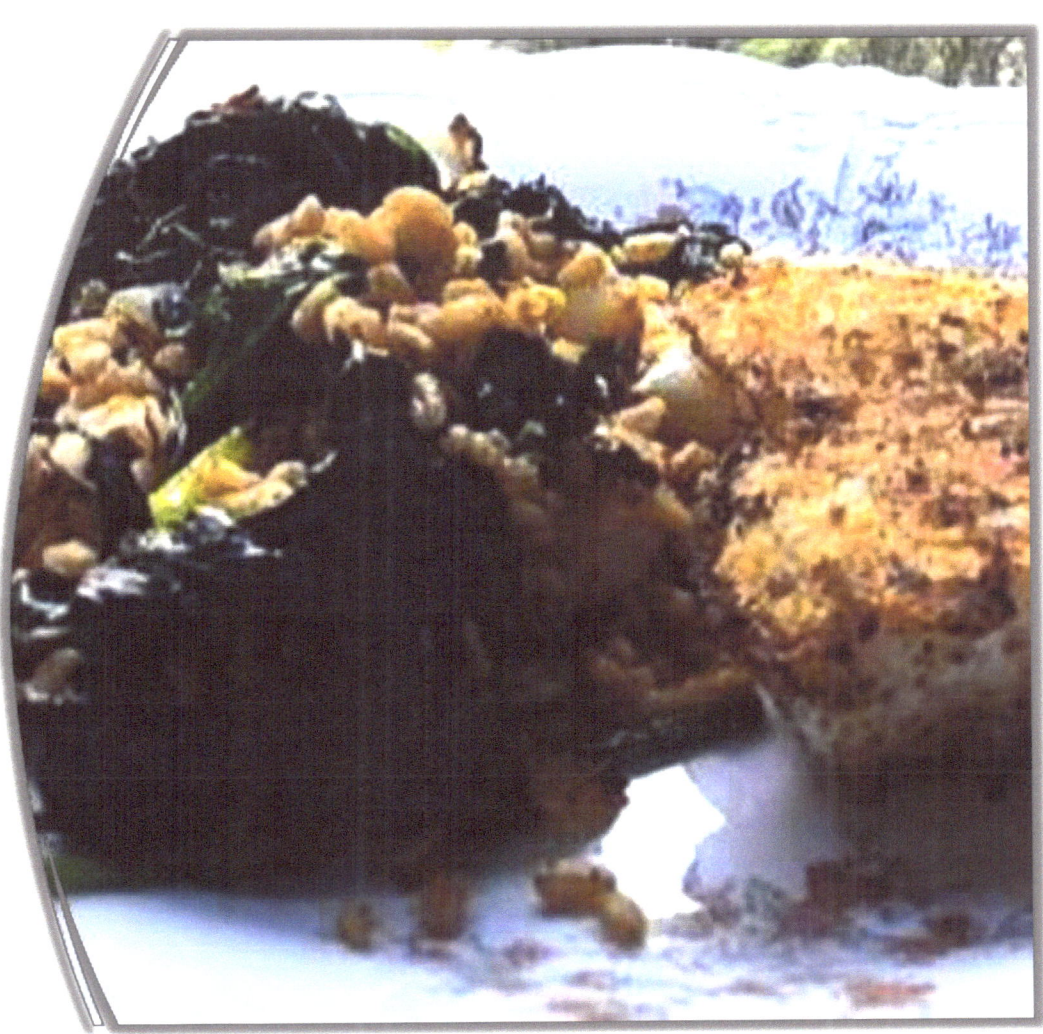

11. COD. PALMETTO. ASPARAGUS

Ingredients:

1 pound of cod or ½ a kilo of any white flaky fish, brushed with olive oil and seasoned with salt and pepper. Grilled for 17 minutes, flip only once.

A bunch or ½ a kilo of asparagus. Cut into mid-size pieces, brushed with olive oil, seasoned with salt and pepper. Grill until you see grill marks on it. Remember to remove the bottom portion (around 1 inch or 2.54 cm) as it tends to be tough

1 can of palmetto, cut into thick pieces.

1 cup of barley or Freekeh boiled and strained.

1 TBSP of mustard.

3 TBSP of olive oil.

Juice of 1 lemon.

Zest of 1 lemon.

Combine and mix all ingredients into a bowl, add the mustard, lemon juice, salt and pepper, 2 TBSP of olive oil, add the zest of 1 lemon.

Serve alongside the grilled fish.

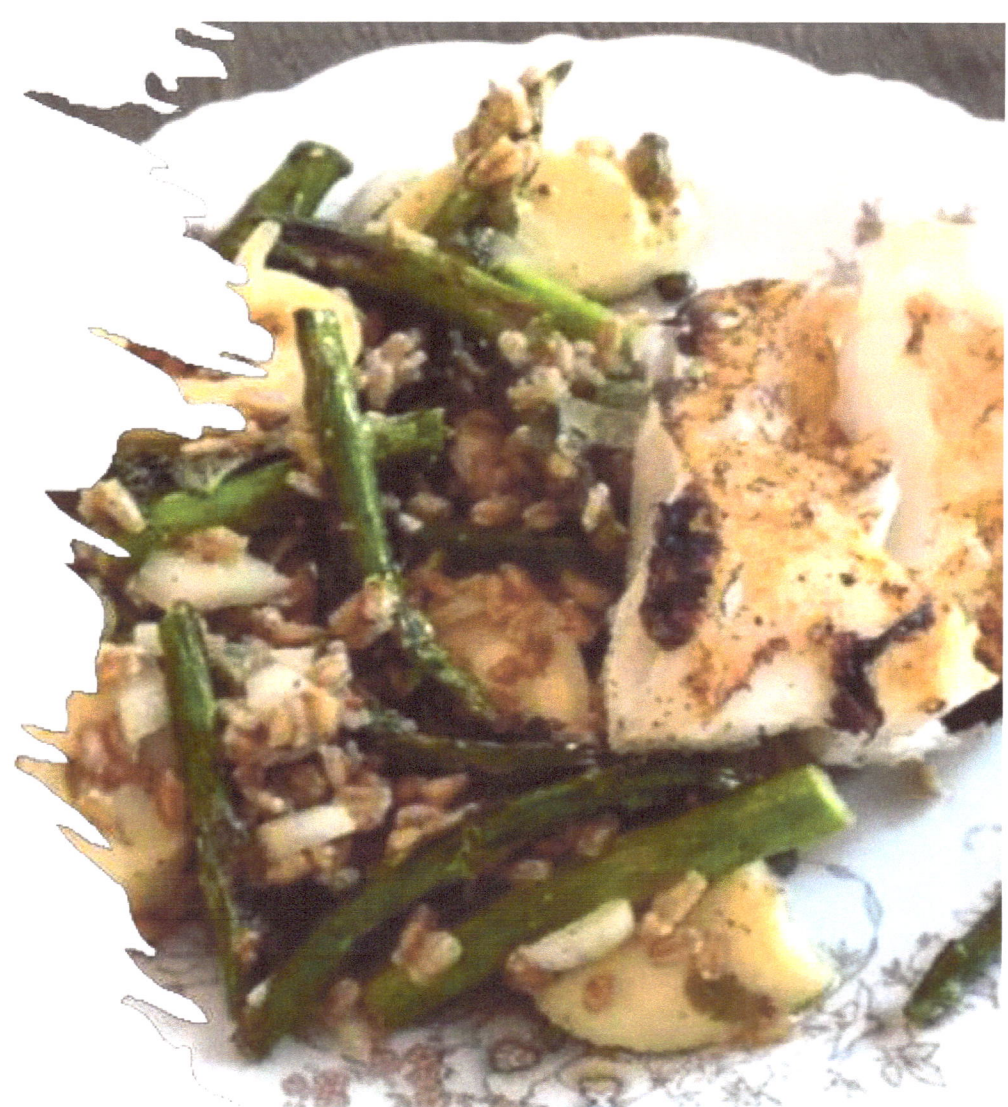

12. COD. POTATO. VEGGIES

Ingredients:
1 Pound of half a kilo of cod or any flaky fish.
Seasoned with salt. Pepper, brushed with olive
oil and Granulated mustard. Grill on medium
heat for 17 minutes, flip only once.
2 cups of sliced grilled colored carrots
½ a diced white onion
A few fresh stems of mint leaves, chopped
1 TSP of granulated mustard
2 tablespoons of olive oil
1 baked potato for each person, seasoned with
salt and pepper, brushed with olive oil, and
baked for 1 hour on medium heat.
Mix all ingredients together.
Serve alongside the grilled fish and baked
potato.

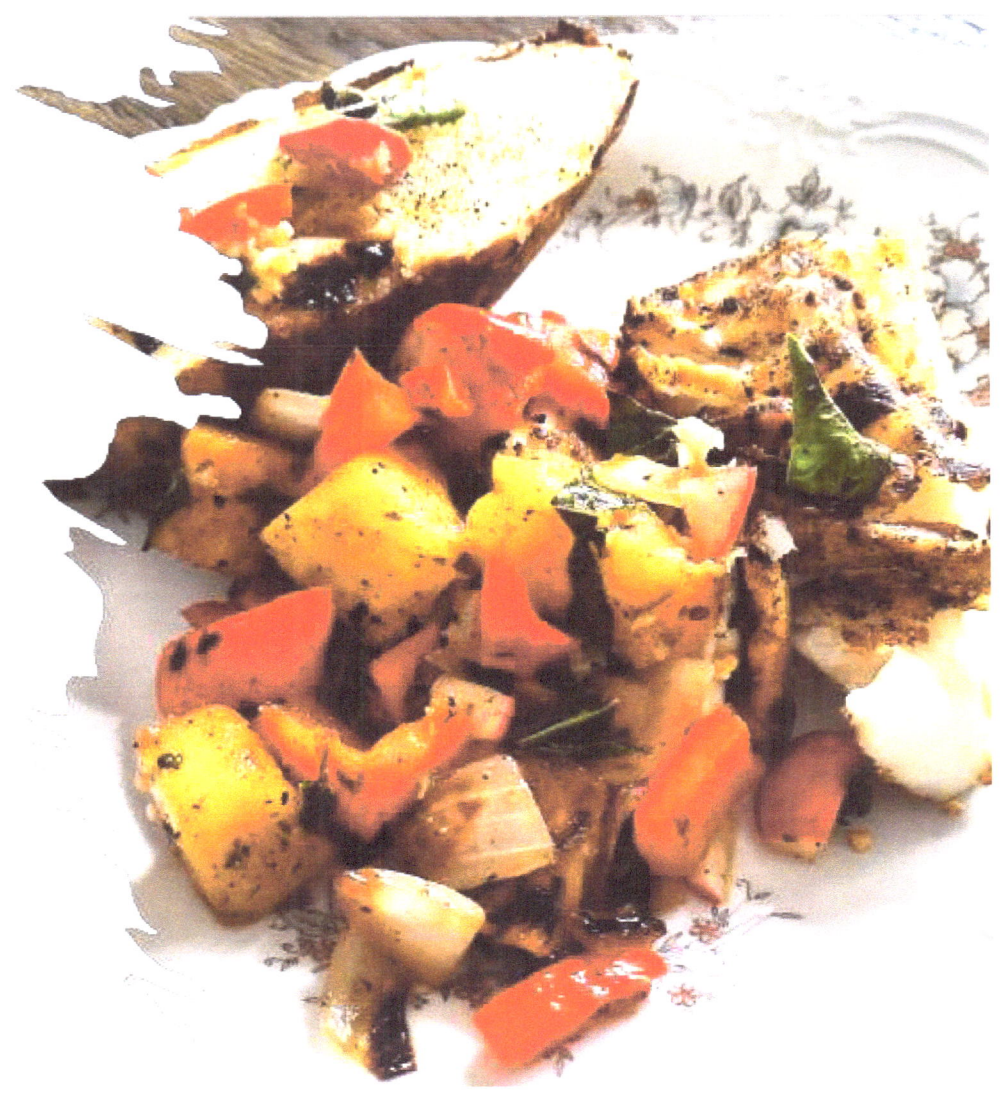

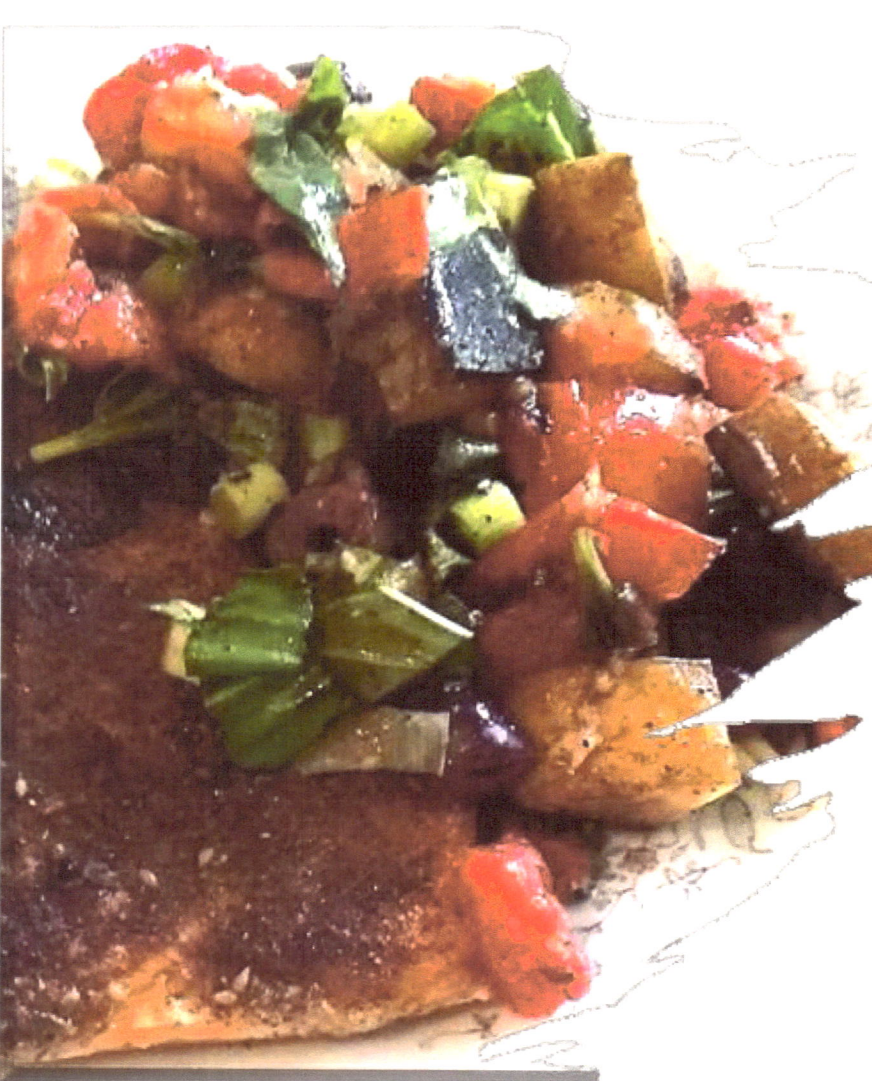

13. SALMON. POTATO. VEGGIES

Ingredients:
1 pound or half a kilo of fresh wild salmon, brushed with olive oil, seasoned with salt and pepper, grilled on medium heat for 19 minutes, flip only once.
1 big-sized tomato or 2 medium-sized ones, chopped into cubes.
Half a head of Romaine lettuce, chopped.
½ a cup of Kalamata olives, chopped.
1 bunch or 6 stems of green onions, chopped
2 TBSP of olive oil
1 TBSP of white vinegar
1 head of potato, cubed, brushed with olive oil, seasoned with salt and pepper, roasted in oven on medium heat for an hour or until it's soft.
Mix all ingredients in a bowl.
Serve alongside the grilled salmon.

14. SHRIMP.
RED ONION. POTATO. MUSTARD

Ingredients:
1 pound or half a kilo of precooked shrimp, brushed with olive oil, seasoned with salt and pepper, grilled for 4 minutes a side
1/4 head of diced red onion
1 TBSP of granulated mustard
2 TBSP of olive oil
1 head of cubed boiled potato.
1 bunch or 6 stems of chopped green onions.
1 TBSP of capers.
Mix all ingredients in a bowl.
Serve alongside the grilled shrimp.

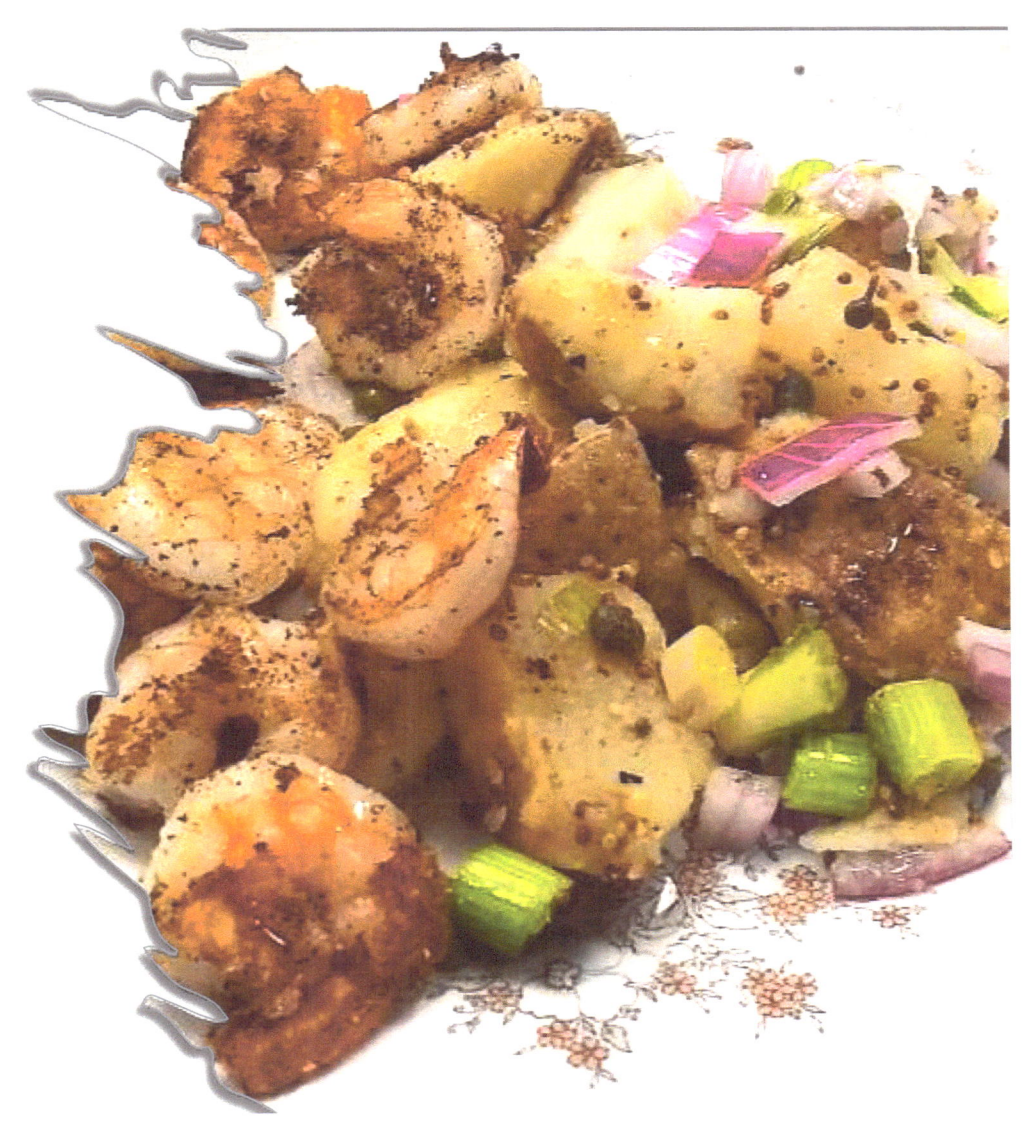

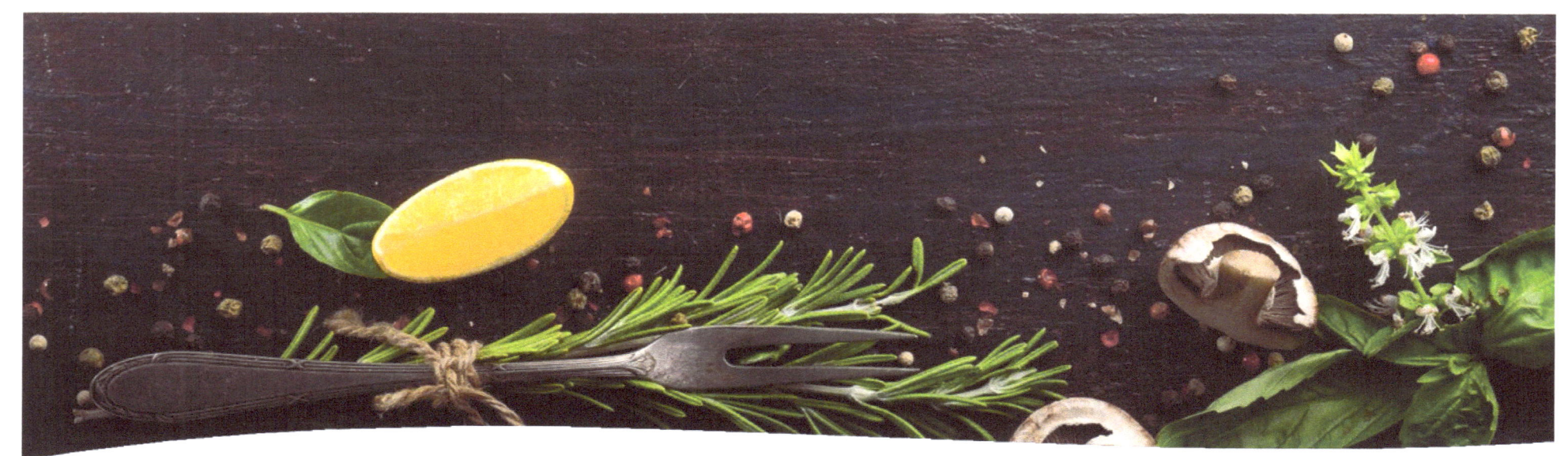

VEGETARIAN

Recipes Mediterranean Inspired

1. BLACK BEANS. SWEET POTATO

Ingredients:

1 cup of boiled and strained pinto beans or black beans.

2 sweet potatoes roasted in the oven for an hour, then cut into big chunks.

1 bunch of cilantro, diced small.

6 stems of green onions, chopped

Slivers of 4 shiitake mushrooms or any available mushrooms. Brushed with oil and seasoned with salt and pepper. Grilled until brown.

3 TBSP of olive oil

Zest and juice of 1 lemon.

Combine and mix all these ingredients in a bowl.

Add the zest and lemon juice, followed by olive oil, salt and pepper.

You can serve this dish by itself as it has protein from the beans or alongside the any seafood or poultry.

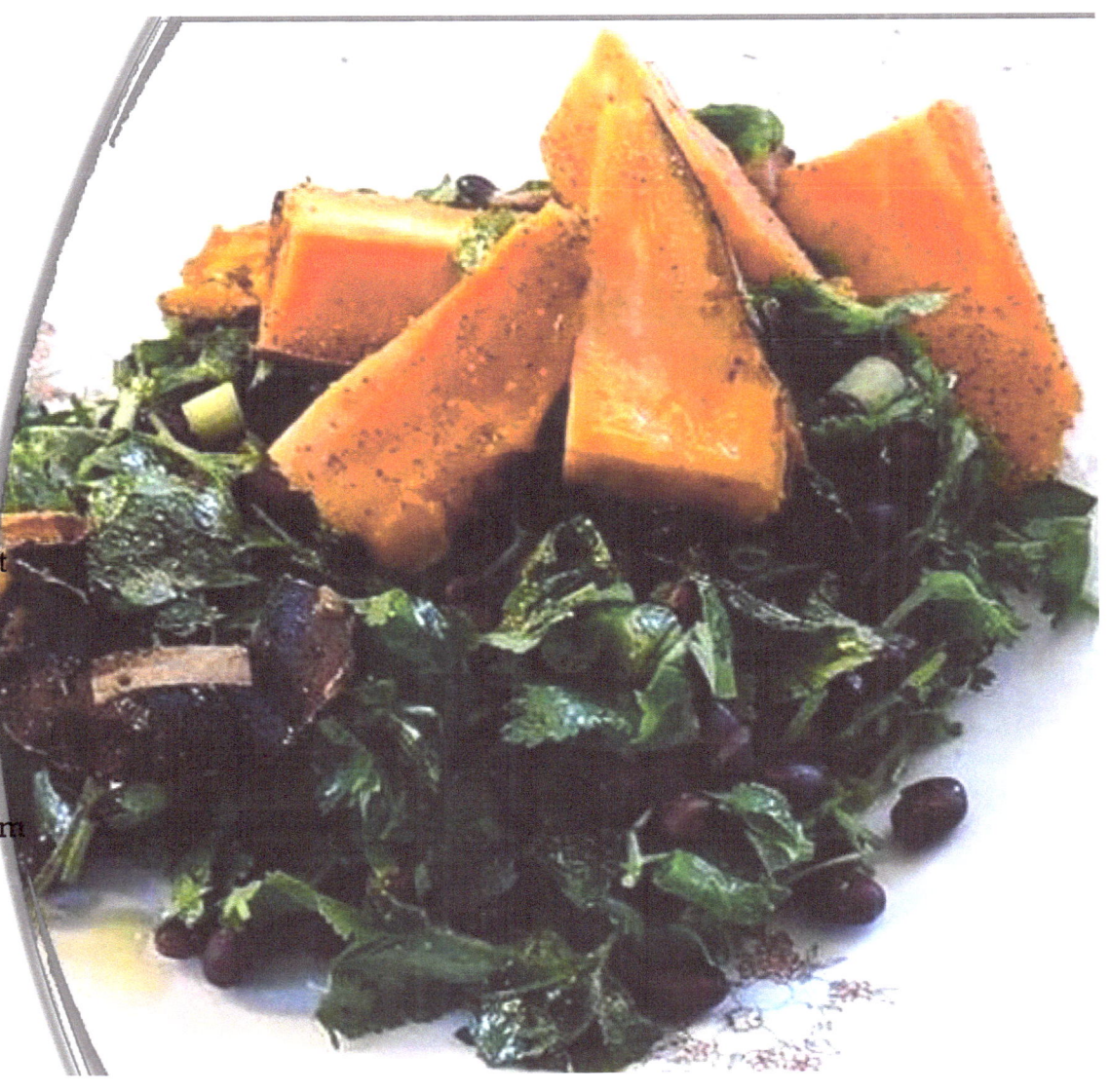

2. KALE. BEANS

Ingredients:
1 cup of boiled and strained red beans.
1 bunch of kale.
1 onion, diced small.
1 lemon juice, zest it before squeezing it.
3 TBSP of sumac.
4 TBSP of olive oil for the cooking of the kale
2 TBSP of olive oil for the whole mix.
Sauté the olive oil with the diced onion; when the onions wilt, add the bunch of kale, sauté, cook until it wilts and shrinks down.
In a bowl, add the boiled beans, the lemon zest and lemon juice, sprinkle with sumac, salt and pepper. You can serve this dish by itself or next to any poultry or seafood.

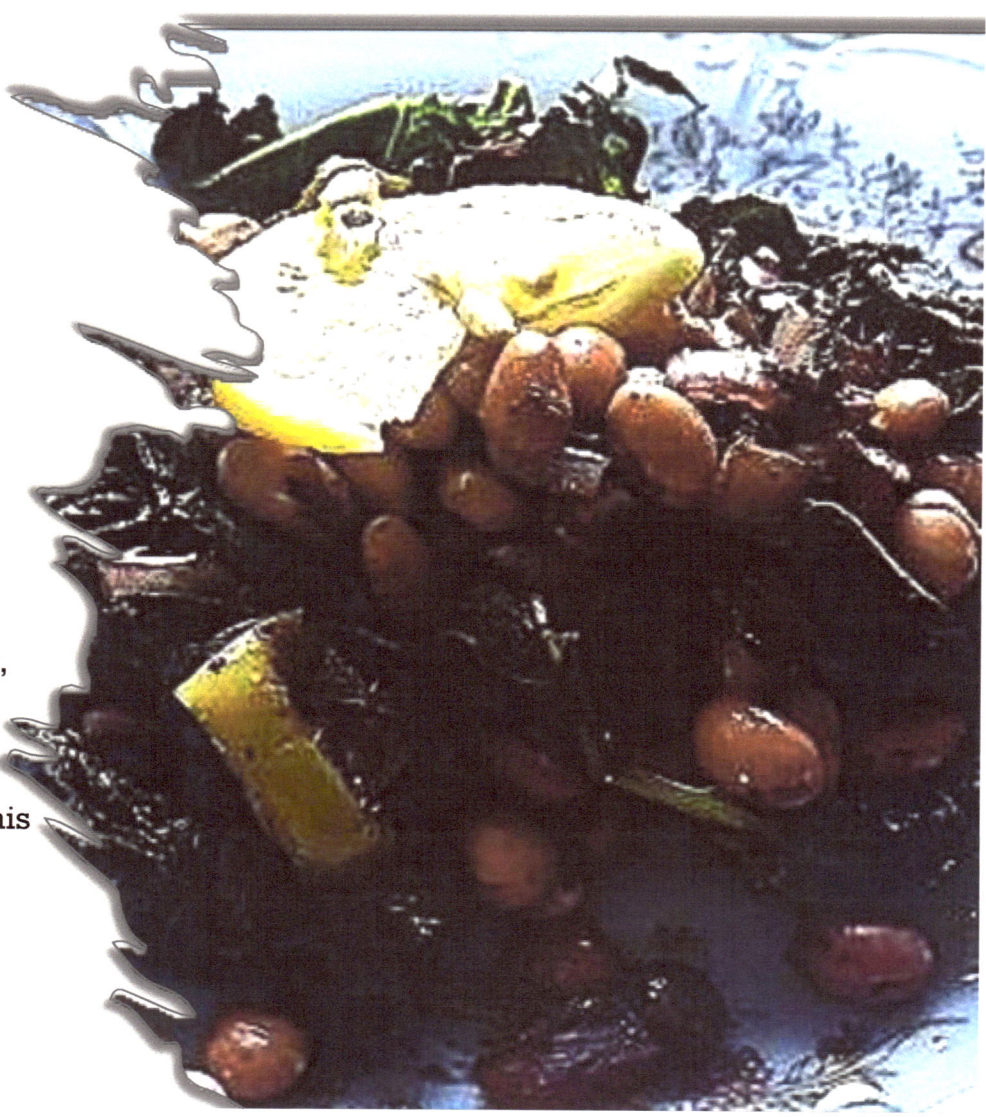

3. ZUCCHINI, LENTILS, ONIONS

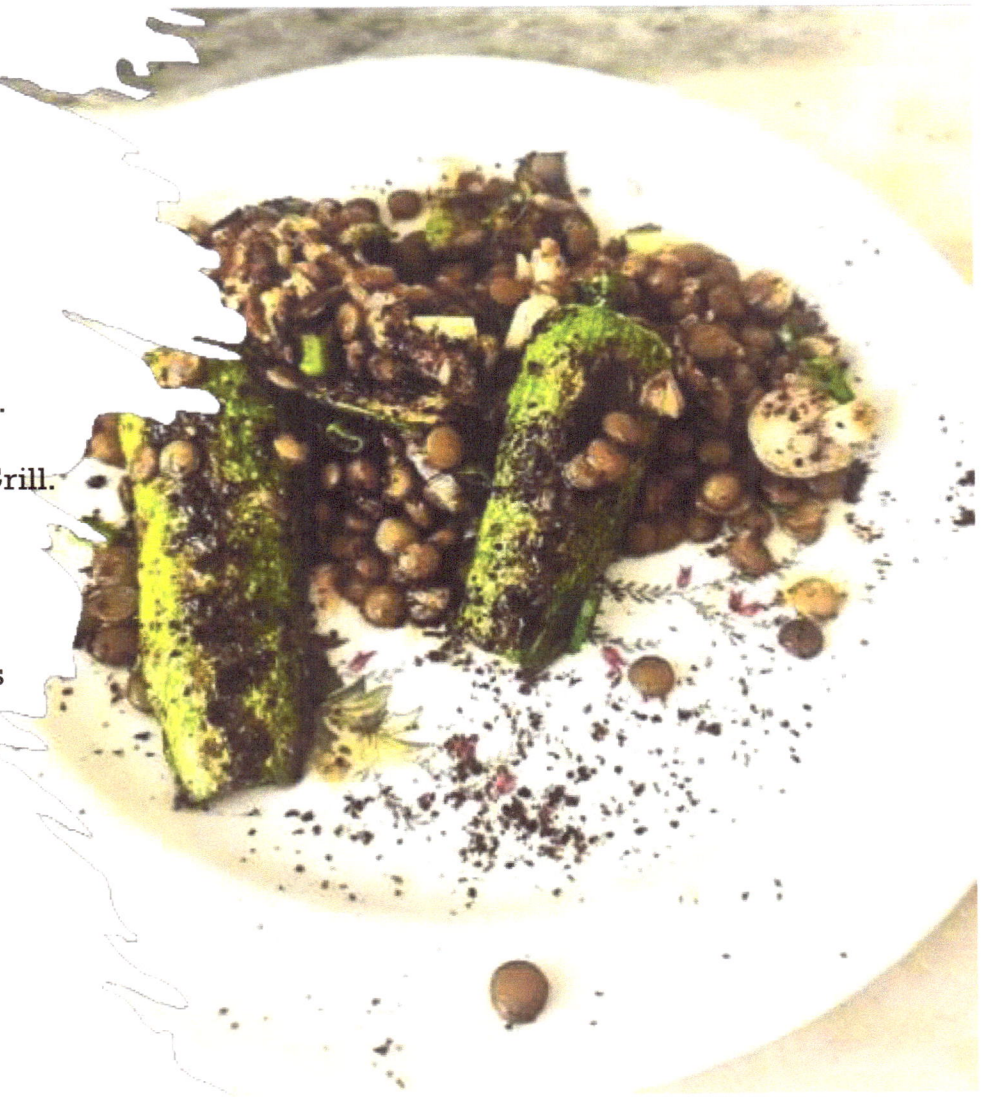

Ingredient:

1 cup of boiled and strained lentils. Any kind of lentils works.
3 Zucchini, mid to small size, sliced into elongated slices,
brushed with olive oil, sprinkled with salt and pepper then Grill.
4 stems of green onions, diced
2 TBSP of olive oil
3 TBSP of sumac
2 diced cloves of garlic
Combine the boiled, strained lentils with diced green onions
with the grilled zucchini in a bowl.
Add the olive oil, sumac, and garlic.
Serve by adding a sprinkle of sumac on top.

4. CAULIFLOWER. OLIVES. WHEAT.

Ingredients:

A big, thick slice of cauliflower for each person. Brushed with olive oil and Dijon mustard, seasoned with salt and pepper, grilled for at least 40 minutes until tender.
Afterward, brown the cauliflower on each side in a pan for added flavor and texture.
½ a cup of Kalamata olives, pitted.
3/4 cup of Wheat boiled and strained.
A few leaves of chopped mint leaves
3 TBSP of olive oil
1 TBSP of Dijon mustard
1 TBSP of capers.
Mix all ingredients in a bowl, season with a pinch of salt and black pepper.
The mix will be served alongside the cauliflower.
You can also serve this dish alongside any grilled or roasted poultry piece or seafood.

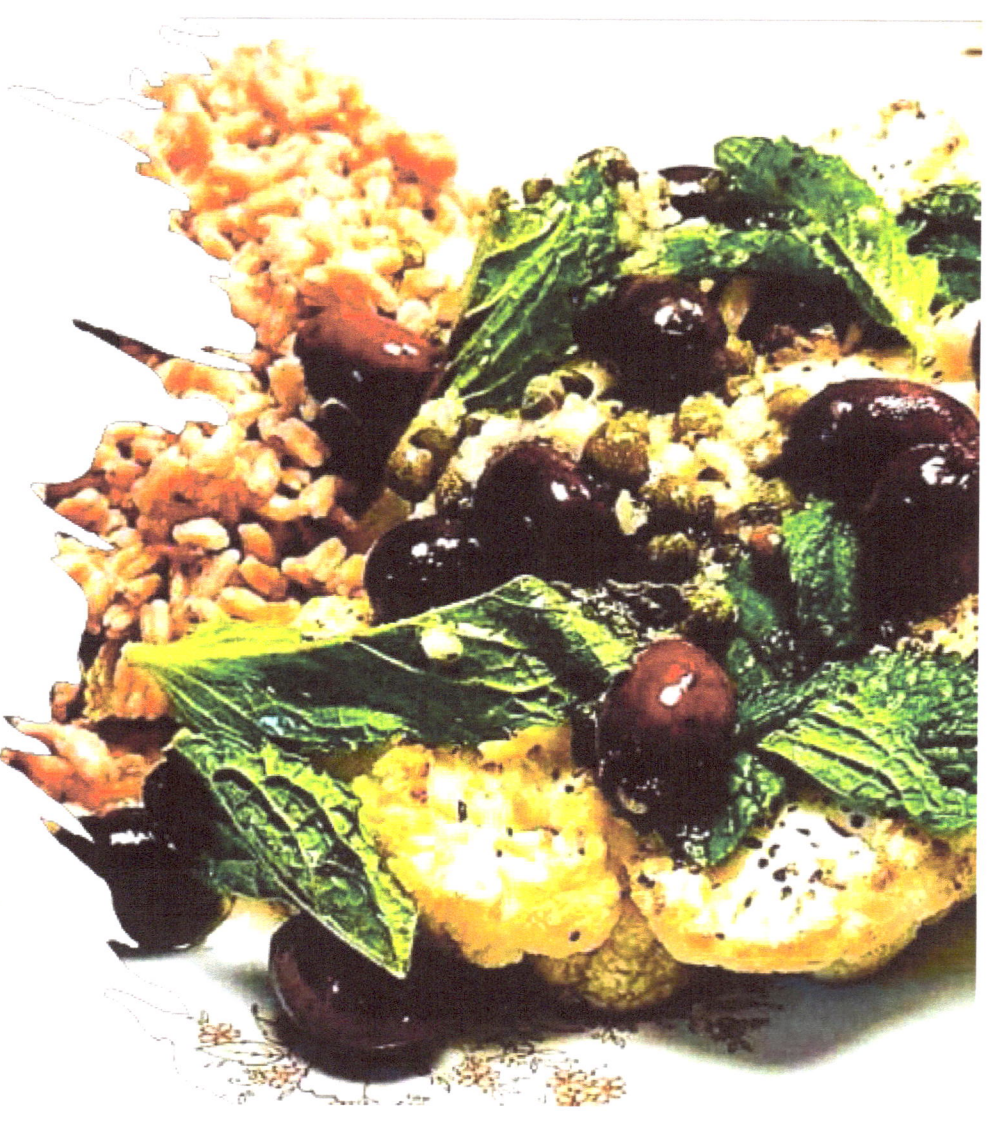

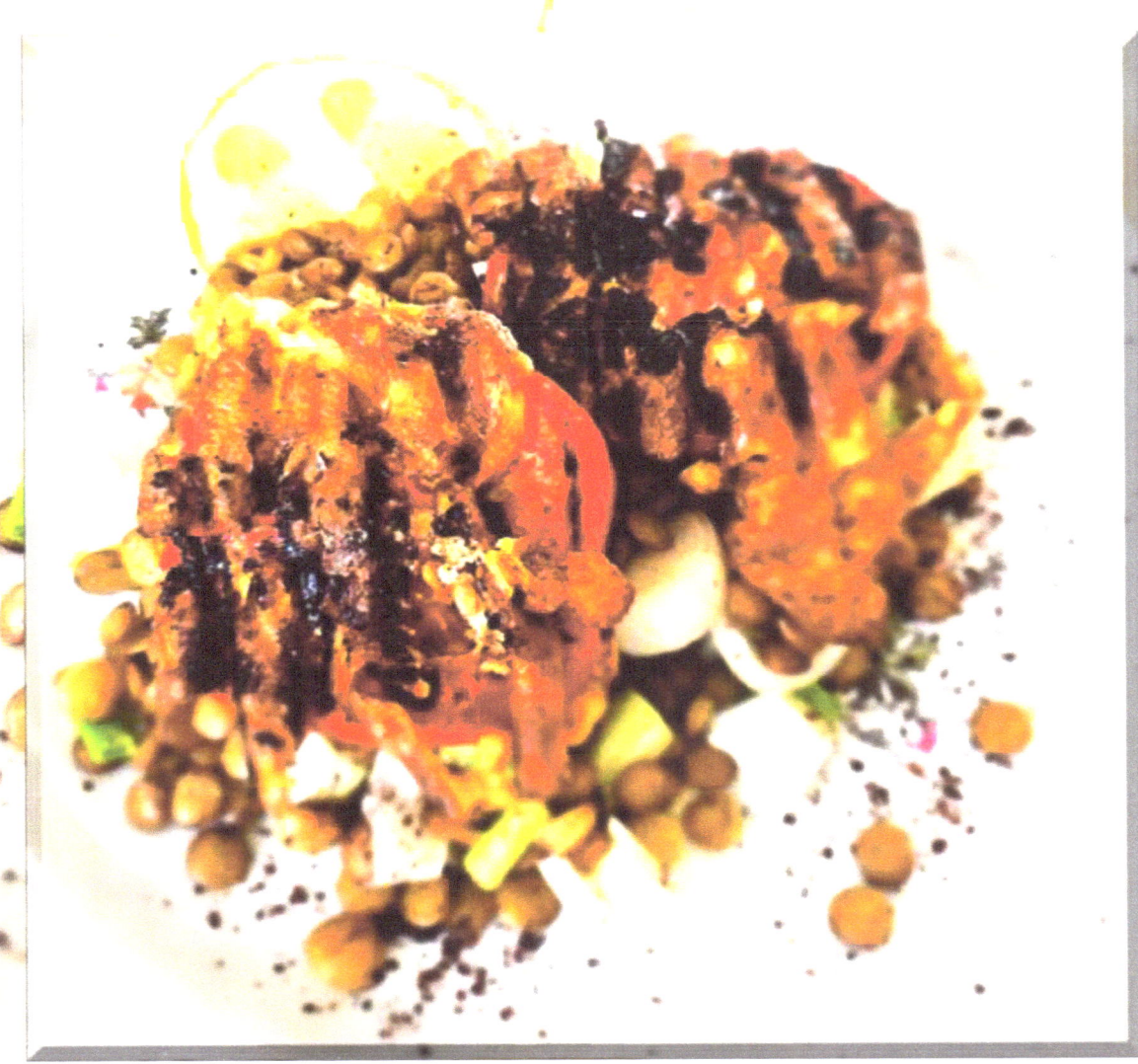

5. LENTILS. TOMATOES. EGGS

Ingredients:
1 cup of lentils, boiled, strained.
6 stems of chopped green onions.
2 mid-size tomatoes, sliced thick, take out the inner part & grill until soft.
Zest and squeeze one lemon.
3 TBSP olive oil.
4 eggs, poured when raw over the middle part of the tomato slices.
Mix all ingredients then place on top of boiled lentils.
Serve this dish by itself or alongside any seafood or poultry

6. EGGPLANT. TOMATO. CHEESE

Ingredients:
2 tomatoes, cut into big chunks, seasoned with salt and pepper, grilled until soft
1 big-size eggplant, cut in half, seasoned with salt and pepper, brushed with olive oil, grilled on medium heat for 44 minutes. Cover for the first 20 minutes.
¼ cup of olive oil.
¼ cup of chopped fresh basil.
1 cup of any shredded cheese, mozzarella, or cheddar.
6 cloves of minced garlic.
¼ cup of chopped olives, green or black.
1 tablespoon of capers.
1 of 15 ounces of tomato sauce.
Mix all ingredients in a bowl, spread the mix on top of the grilled eggplant in an oven pan.
Pour the shredded cheese on top of all.
Pan goes in the oven on medium heat for 12 minutes or 14 minutes, or until the cheese is melted.
You can always enhance this dish by adding roasted or grilled shredded chicken.

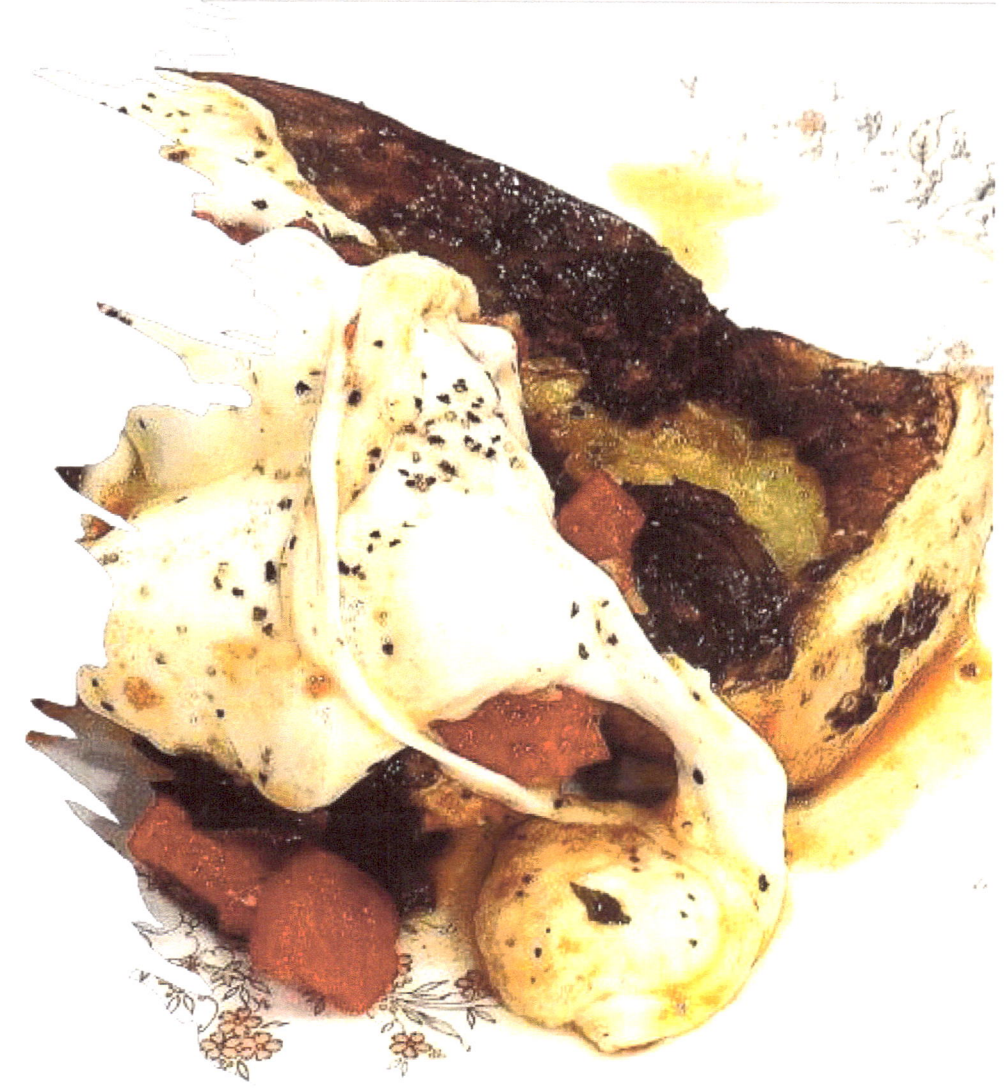

7. LENTILS. SWEET POTATO

Ingredients:
1 cup of boiled lentils, strained; any kind of lentils works.
1 head of decent-sized sweet potato cut into thick slices,
seasoned with salt and pepper, brushed with olive oil,
grilled or roasted in oven on medium heat for an hour.
½ a cup of crumbled feta cheese.
Half a bunch of chopped parsley
4 cloves of minced garlic
½ an onion chopped fine.
¼ cup of olive oil
Zest and a squeeze of one lemon
Mix all ingredients in a bowl, add the feta cheese on top.
You can always have this dish by itself or alongside any
poultry or grilled seafood.

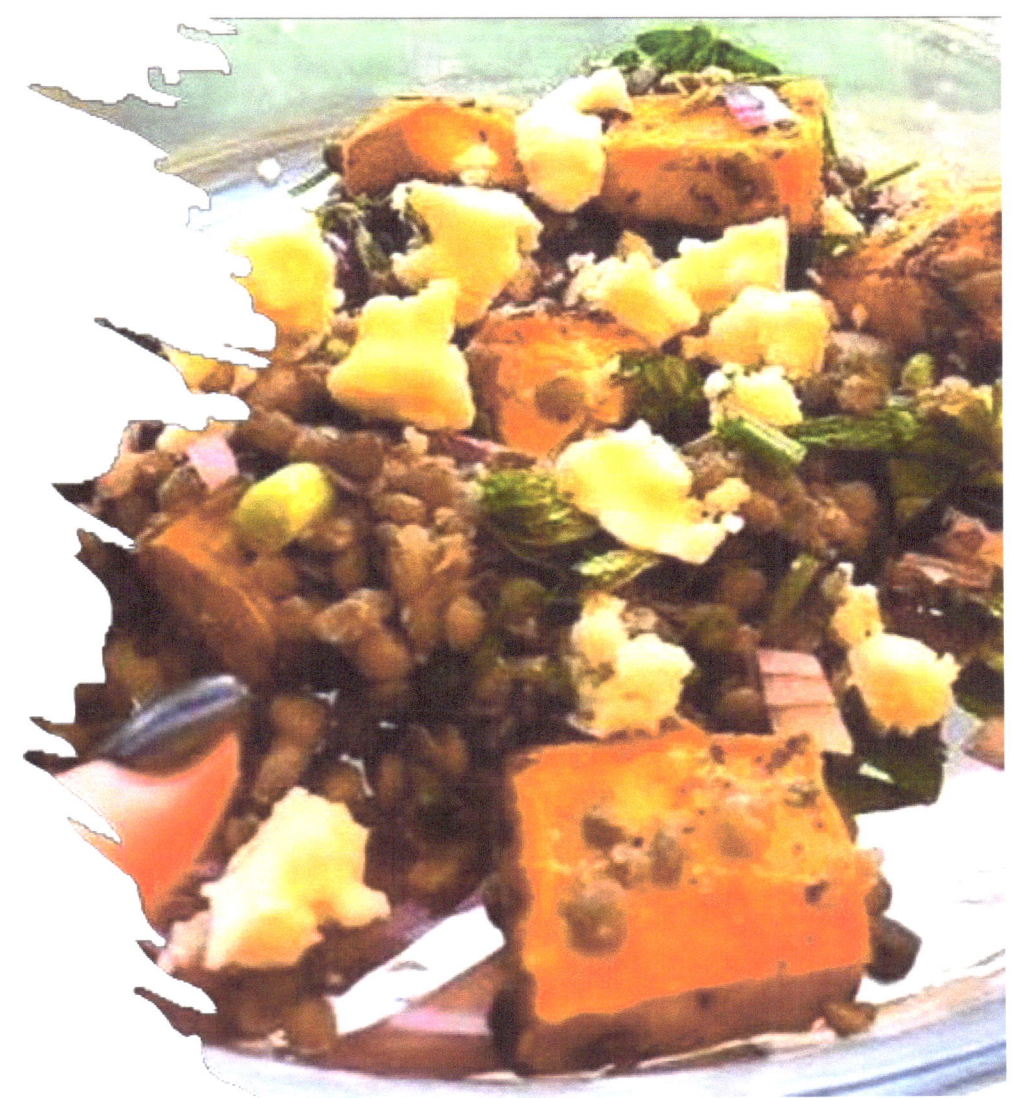

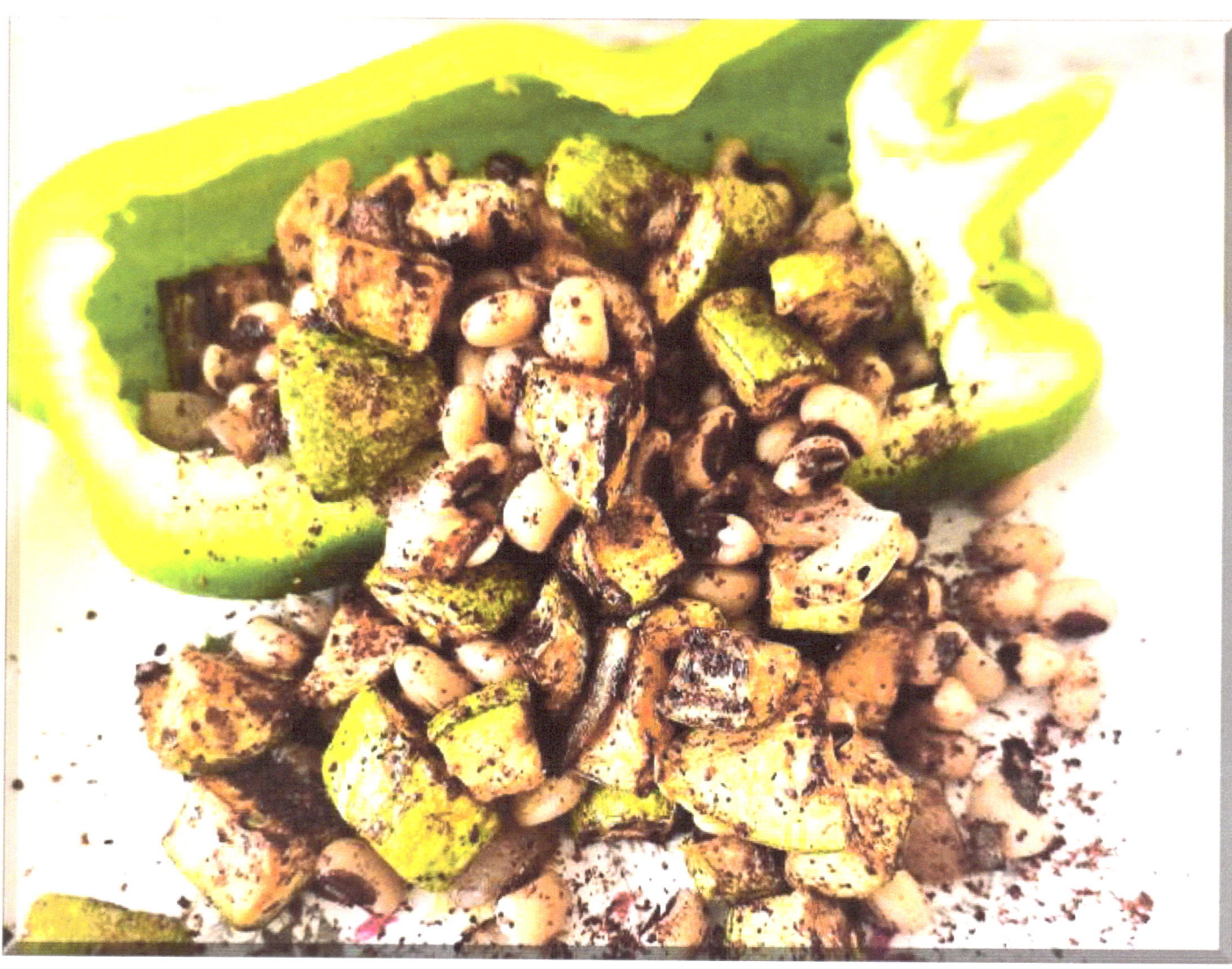

8. GREEN PEPPER. ZUCCHINI. BEANS

Ingredients:

One green pepper cut in half

2 cubed Zucchinis, salted and peppered then grilled.

1/2 Grilled diced red onion

1 TBL sumac

2 TBL of olive oil.

3/4 cup of boiled and strained black eyed peas

Mix all and place the mix on top of the green pepper.

Recipes Mediterranean Inspired

9. GREEN BEANS. CHICKPEAS

Ingredients:

½ a cup of chickpeas, boiled, strained.

1 pound of green beans, cut into big.

1 medium-sized onion, diced small.

1 chopped green pepper.

Sprinkle 1 TSP of garlic powder, cayenne pepper, salt, pepper.

1 TBLS of sumac.

Add a small amount of olive oil to the onions, and sauté until they wilt. Then add the green beans to the wilted onions and sauté for 5 minutes, add 1 cup of water, cover, and let it simmer for 25 minutes on low heat.

Once the green beans are done, add to the chickpeas and chopped green pepper, sprinkle all with sumac.

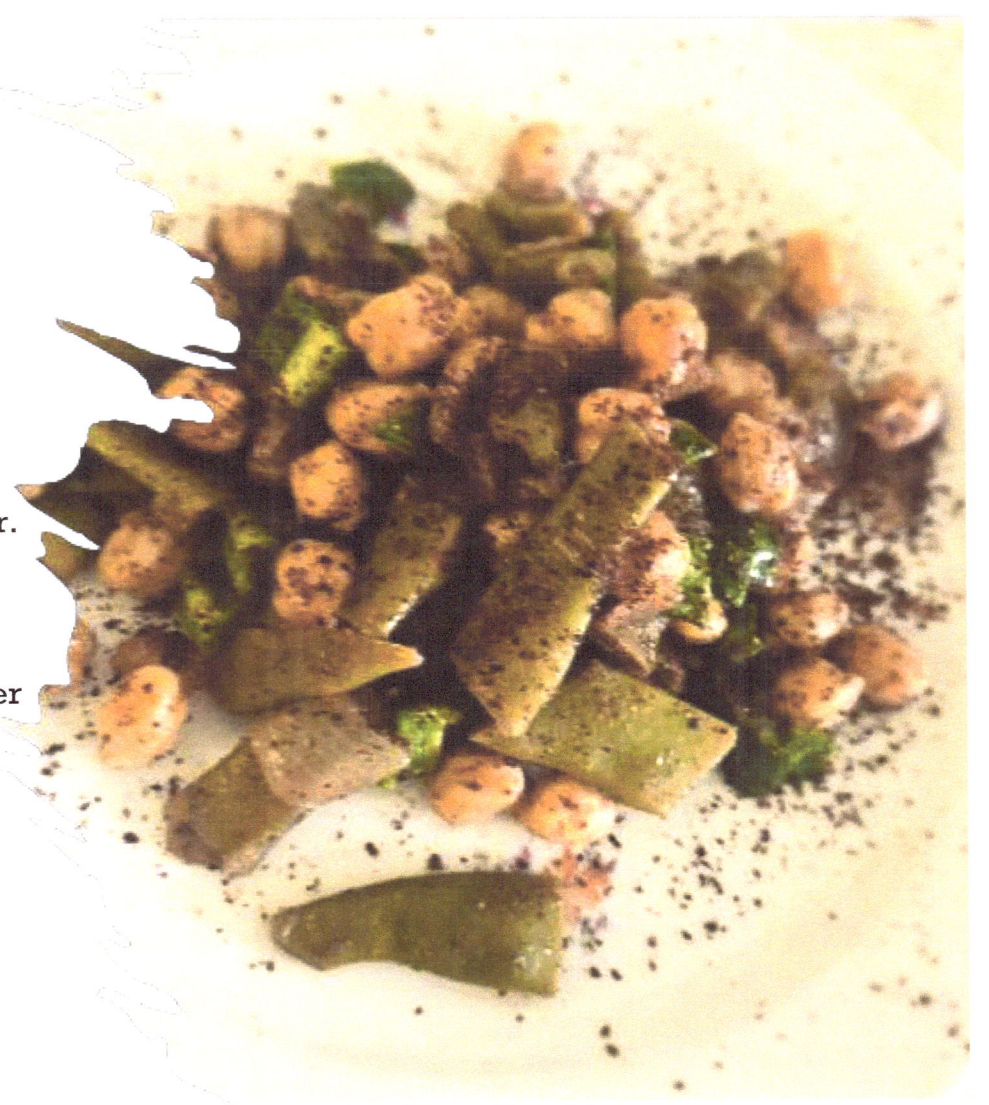

POULTRY

Recipes Mediterranean Inspired

1. WATERMELON, CHICKEN. WHEAT.

Ingredients:
2 slices of watermelon, cut each into a moon shape.
2 chicken boneless thighs, brushed with olive oil, seasoned with salt and pepper, grilled for around 24 minutes on medium heat, flip only once.
¼ cup of crumbled feta cheese.
¾ cup of wheat or barley, boiled and strained.
6 stems of green onions, small diced.
Zest of 1 lemon.
1 TBSP of olive oil.
1 TBSP of balsamic vinegar.
Combine all ingredients and serve on top of watermelon.

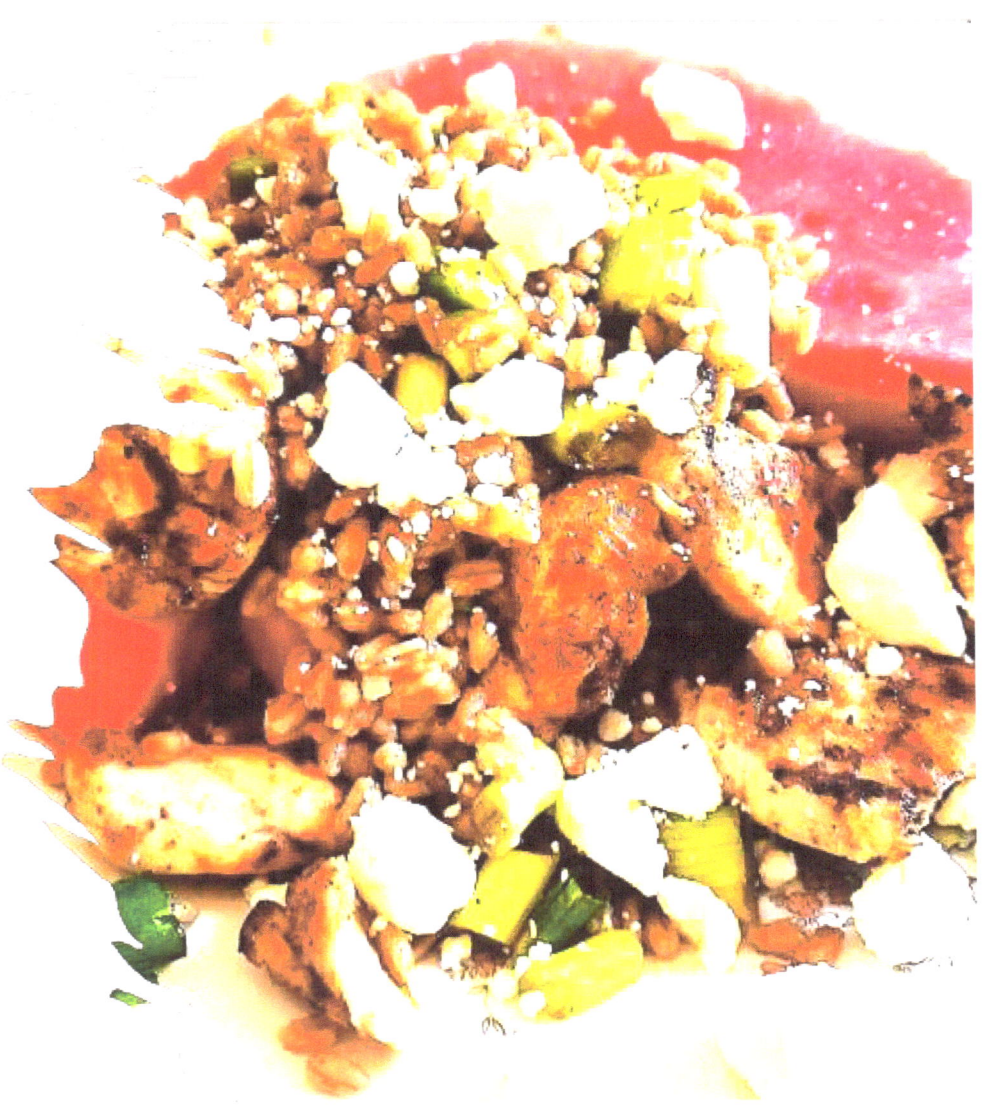

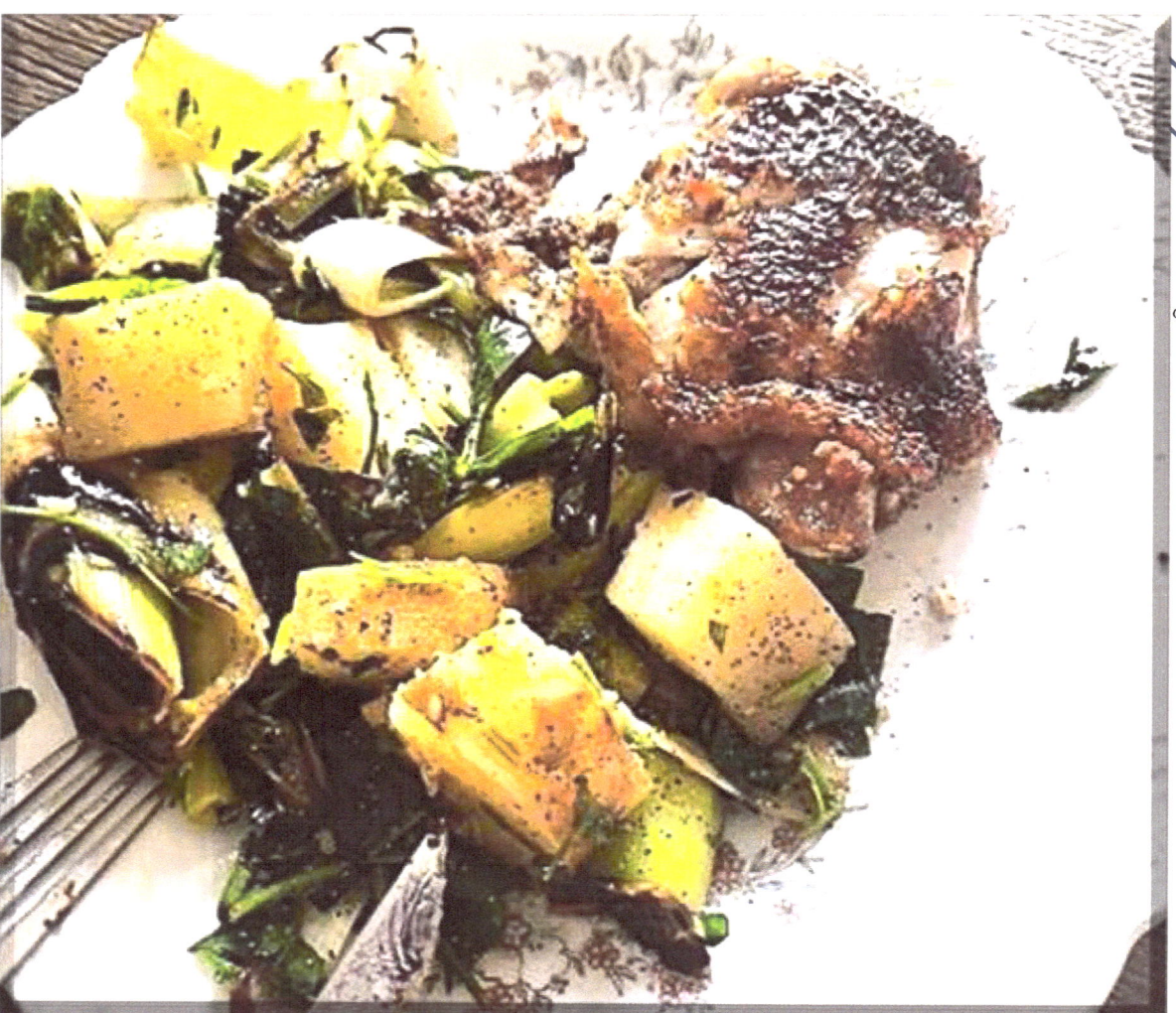

2. CHICKEN, LEEKS.

Ingredients:
2 mid-size potatoes boiled in cubes.
1 bunch of leeks, diced and grilled
2 Thighs of in-bone chicken rubbed with 4 teaspoons of coriander, salt, pepper, and olive oil
A few stems of chopped parsley
1 lemon juiced.
2 TBL olive oil
½ teaspoon of dried coriander
2 cloves of garlic, chopped.
Grill chicken for 40 minutes on medium heat, flipping only once
Combine, the grilled diced leeks and garlic with the boiled potatoes in a bowl.
Add the lemon juice, 2 TBSP olive oil, and ¼ teaspoon of coriander mix.
Add the fresh chopped parsley on top.
Mix all together
Serve this mixture alongside the chicken.

3. CHICKEN. WILD RICE. APRICOT

Ingredients:

2 baby chickens, washed inside out, brushed with 2 tablespoons of olive oil, seasoned with salt and pepper.

½ a cup of slivered almonds

½ a cup of dried apricots cut into small pieces

½ a cup of cooked wild rice

1 head of garlic, peeled and diced

1 tablespoon of Zaatar or dried oregano.

4 tablespoons of olive oil

The zest of a lemon and the juice of one lemon

Combine in a bowl the already cooked rice with chopped apricots, the 2 tablespoons of olive oil, garlic, salt and pepper. The Zest and lemon juice.

Dry the baby chicken completely, then stuff it with the rice and apricot mix.

Tie the legs of the chicken together with cooking yarn, place the chicken on a tray, and brush with olive oil, salt and pepper.

Wrap them in aluminum foil roast them on medium heat for an hour,

Add the almonds on top of the chicken

Put back to the oven for an extra 12 minutes or until the almonds turn to honey color.

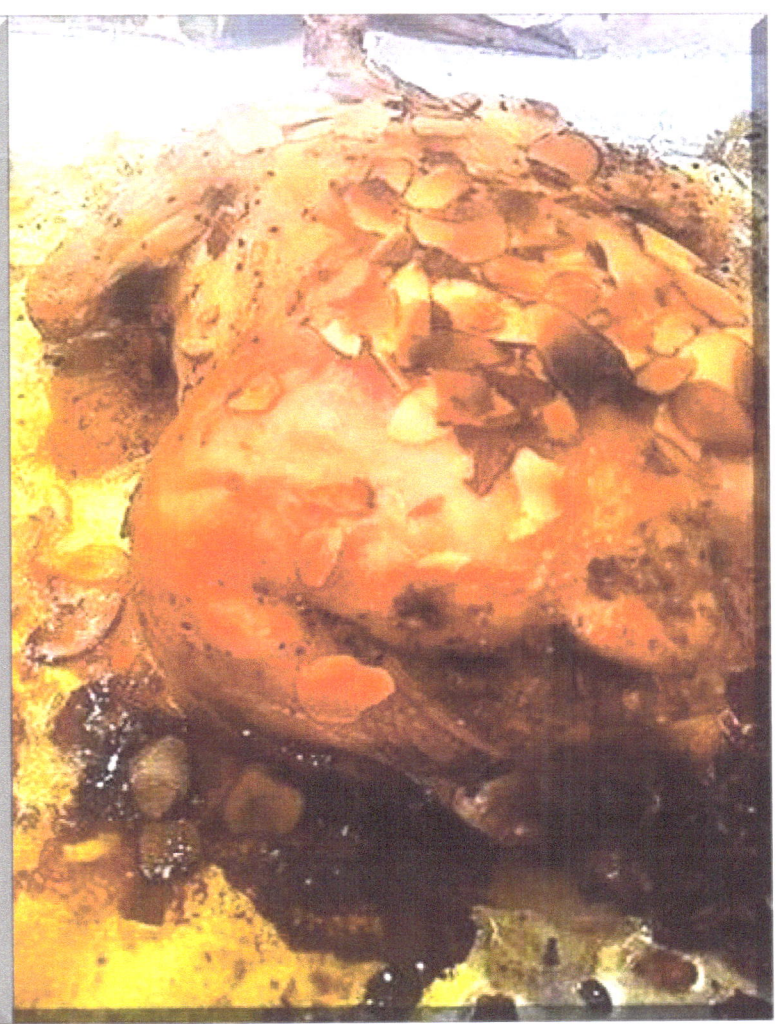

4. CHICKEN. FREEKEH. BROCCOLI

Ingredients:

1 pound or a half kilo of boneless chicken, cut into chunks, marinated for at least an hour with 1 teaspoon of paprika, 2 tablespoons of olive oil, ¼ cup of white vinegar, one head of garlic peeled and minced, a pinch of salt, 1 teaspoon of shish Taouk spice (found in Mediterranean store).

Grill for 8 minutes on medium heat

¾ cup of Freekeh boiled and strained

¼ cup of frozen peas and carrots

4 stems of broccoli, seasoned with salt and pepper, grilled

¼ cup of white vinegar

2 tablespoons of olive oil.

Combine all ingredients, add ¼ cup of white vinegar and 2 tablespoons of olive oil.

Season with a pinch of salt and pepper.

Serve alongside the chicken or shish Taouk.

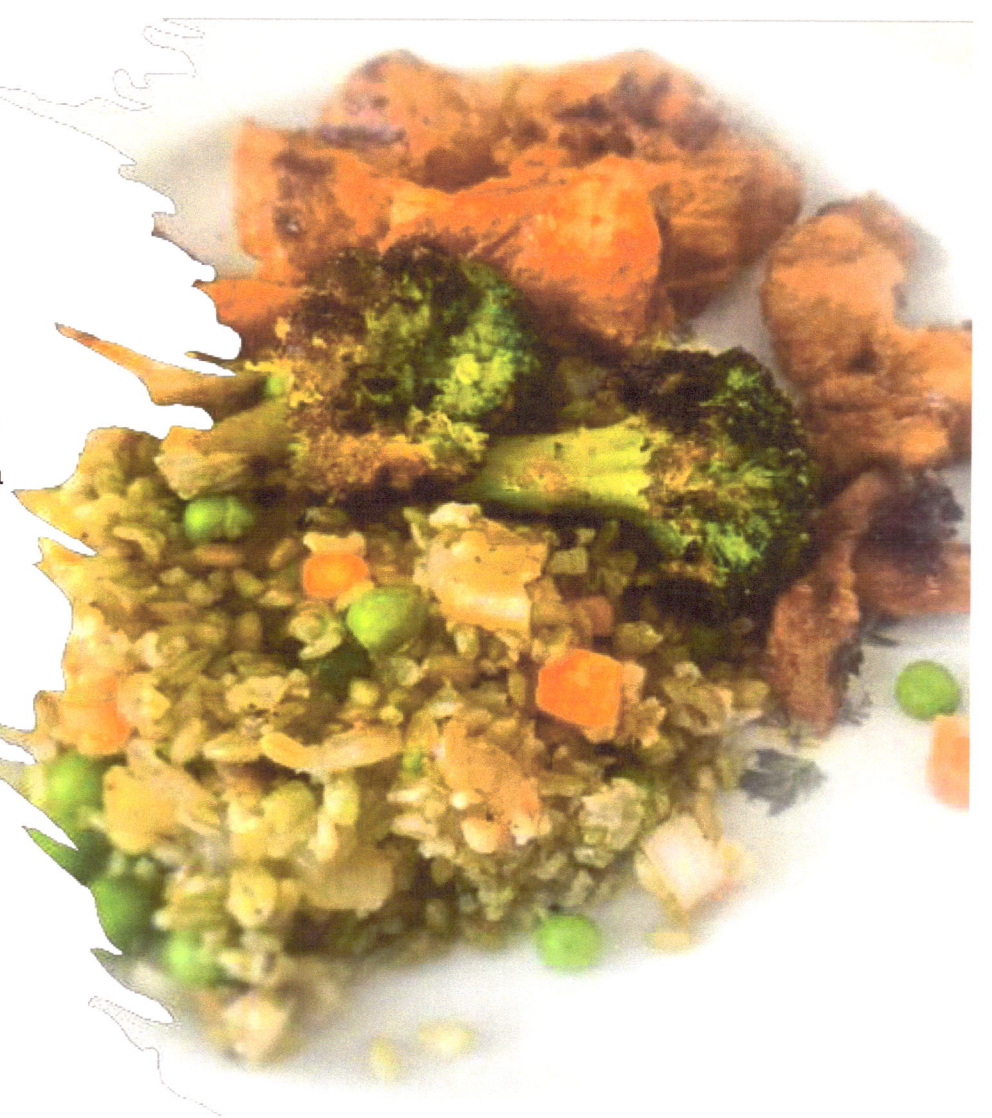

5. CHICKEN. GREEN BEANS

Ingredients:
½ a kilo or 1 pound of salted, peppered, grilled green beans
2 Thighs of boneless chicken, brushed with olive oil, seasoned with salt and pepper, and mustard, grilled for around 24 minutes on medium heat.
½ white onion, diced small.
1 tablespoon granulated mustard for the mix.
2 tablespoons of olive oil.
1 tablespoon of Dijon mustard for chicken.
2 tablespoons of green olives, pitted.
Combine all ingredients and serve alongside the grilled chicken.

.

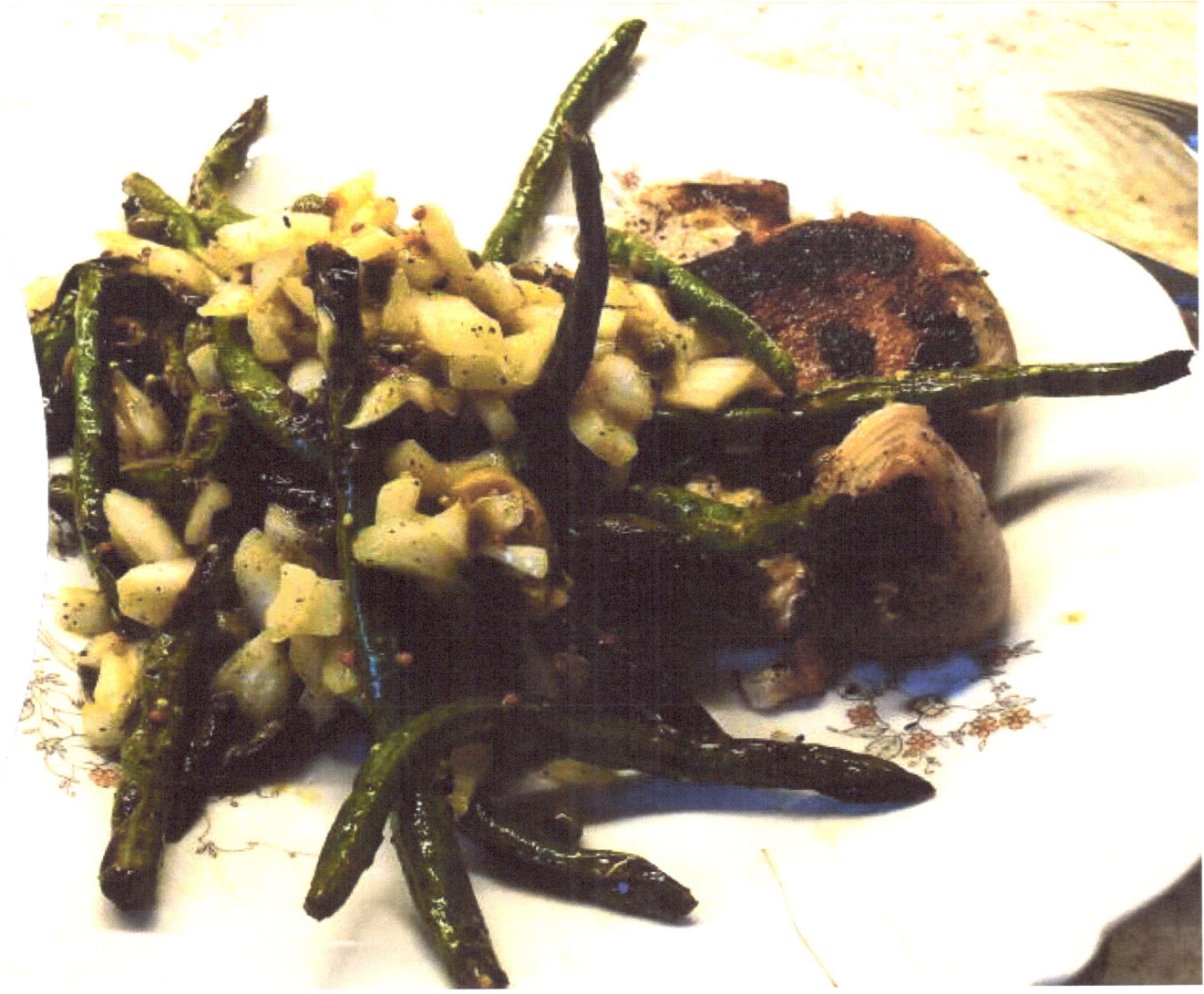

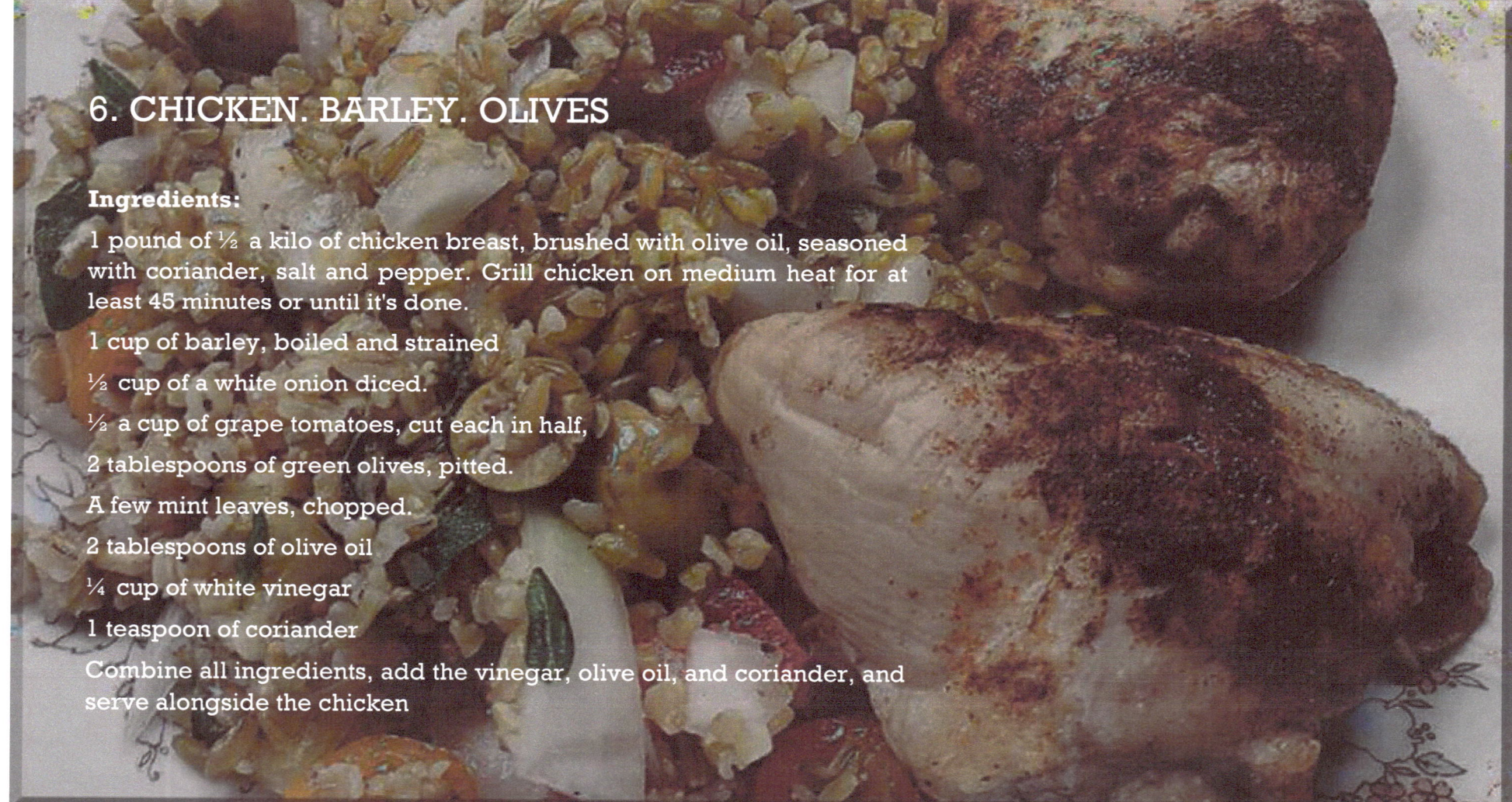

6. CHICKEN. BARLEY. OLIVES

Ingredients:

1 pound of ½ a kilo of chicken breast, brushed with olive oil, seasoned with coriander, salt and pepper. Grill chicken on medium heat for at least 45 minutes or until it's done.

1 cup of barley, boiled and strained

½ cup of a white onion diced.

½ a cup of grape tomatoes, cut each in half,

2 tablespoons of green olives, pitted.

A few mint leaves, chopped.

2 tablespoons of olive oil

¼ cup of white vinegar

1 teaspoon of coriander

Combine all ingredients, add the vinegar, olive oil, and coriander, and serve alongside the chicken

Recipes Mediterranean Inspired

7. CHICKEN. LETTUCE. EGGPLANT. BULGUR

Ingredients:

Use Iceberg lettuce and peel 3 leaves for each person.

Cube one eggplant, brush with olive oil, season with salt and pepper, put in the oven for around 40 minutes on medium heat or until they are soft and done

½ a cup of boiled barley, strained

2 tablespoons of soy sauce

¼ cup of rice vinegar

1 tablespoon of sesame seeds

6 stems of chopped green onion

Season the chicken with salt and pepper, brush with olive oil. Roast the chicken thighs in the oven over medium heat for 45 minutes. Shred the chicken when it's done.

Add the shredded chicken to the mix of all ingredients above

All the mix goes into the lettuce leaves. Serve, and enjoy.

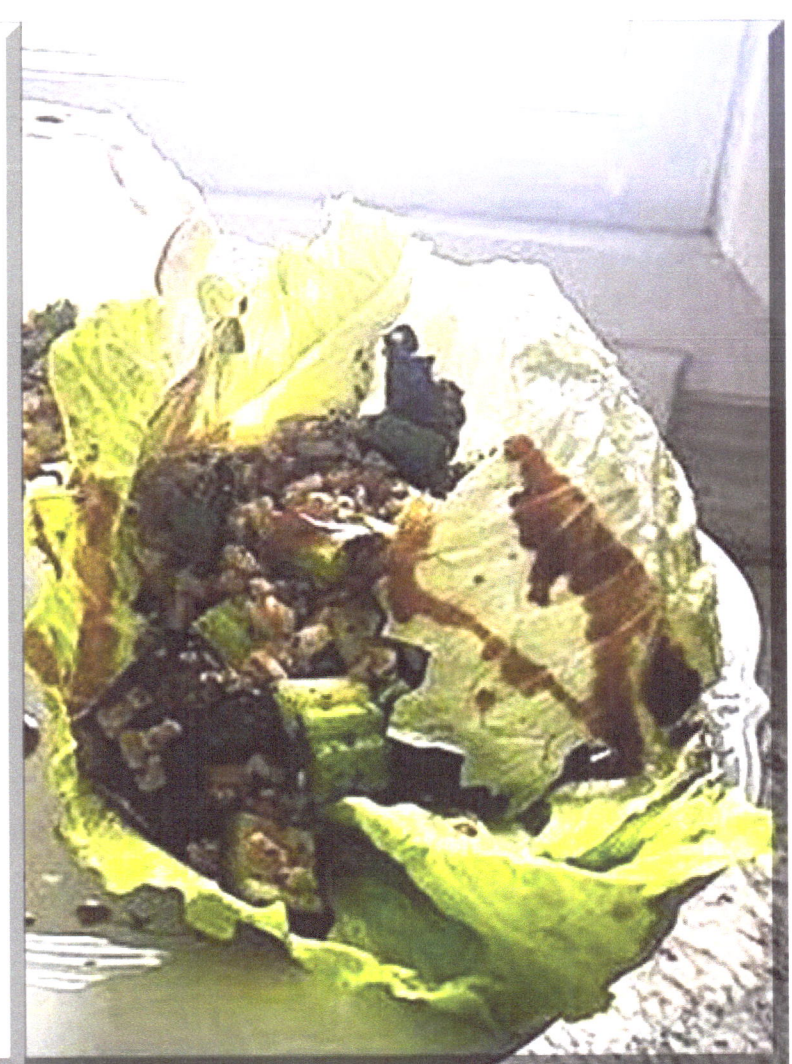

8. CHICKEN BALLS. BLACK-EYED PEAS. SPINACH

Ingredients:

1 pound or ½ kilo of ground chicken, add to it one egg, ¼ cup of breadcrumbs, salt and pepper. Make chicken balls and brush them with olive oil.

Grill the balls on medium heat for 25 minutes or until they're cooked completely.

1 bunch of spinach or 1 pound.

¾ cup of black-eyed peas, boiled and strained

1 onion, diced small.

Zest and juice of 1 lemon

1 tablespoon of sumac

Add the diced onion and 3 tablespoons of olive oil to a pan, sauté until it's wilted, add spinach to the wilted onions. Keep sautéing the mix until spinach wilts.

Add sumac, zest and juice of one lemon.

Serve the mixture alongside the chicken balls.

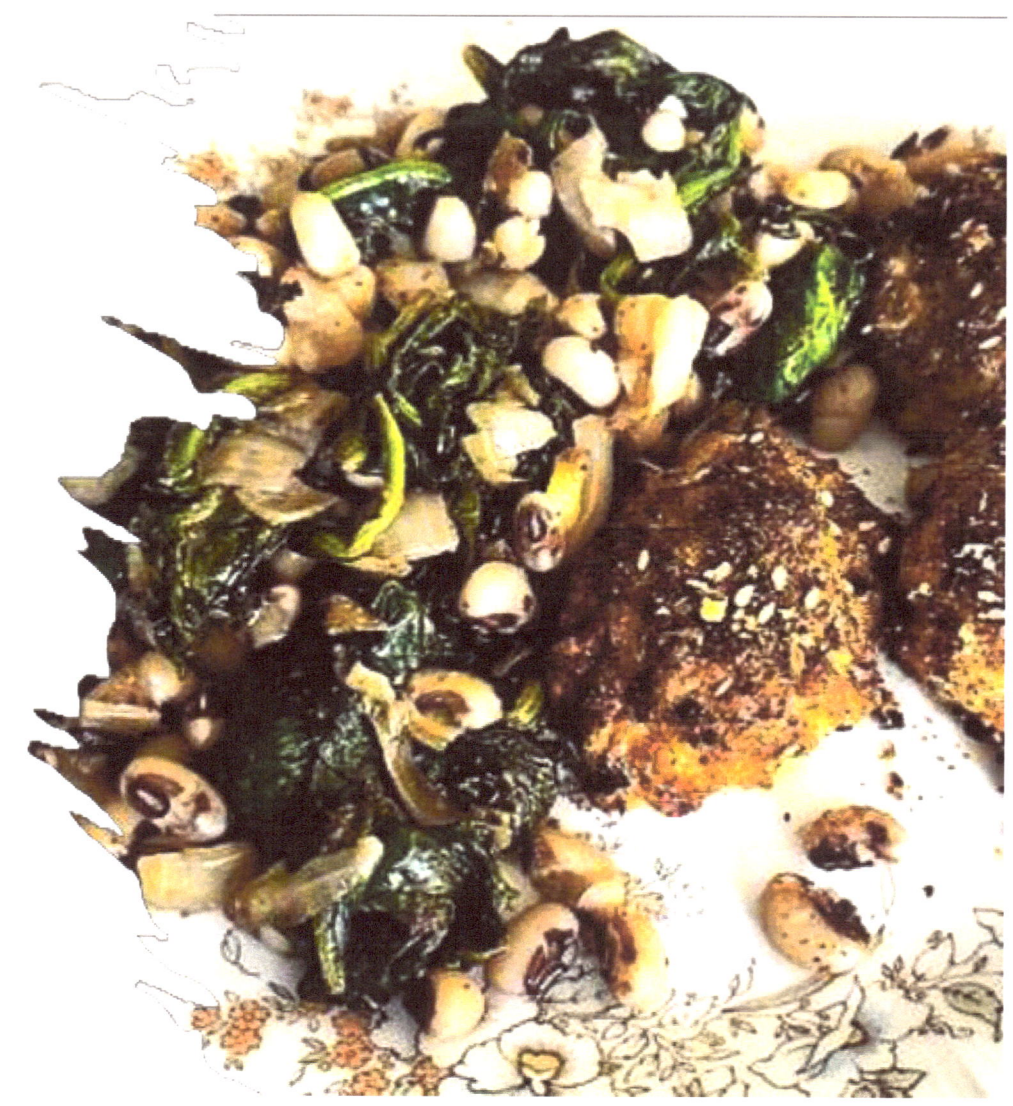

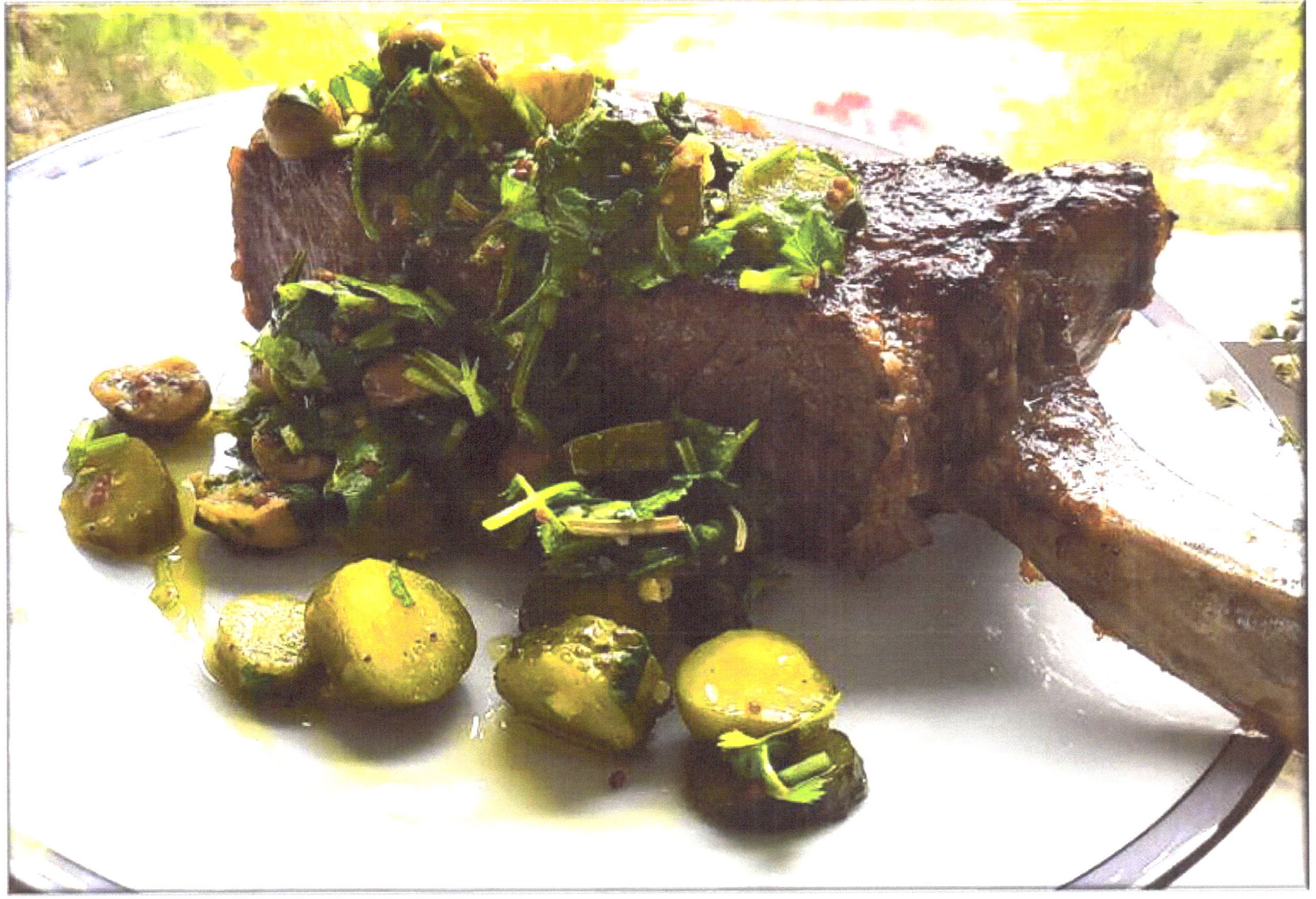

BEEF

1. KOFTA. FREEKEH. ASPARAGUS

Ingredients:

Combine and shape 1 pound or half a kilo of ground beef into finger shape mixed with 1/2 TBSP of harissa, chopped of 1 onion, salt, pepper, and a few stems of chopped parsley.

Grill 1 bunch of asparagus after adding to them olive oil salt and pepper for 16 minutes, flipping them once after 10 minutes.

¾ cup of Freekeh boiled and strained.

½ onion chopped and mixed with Freekeh.

Drizzle of olive oil and white vinegar.

Grill the Kofta on medium heat for 6 minutes each side.

Mix all ingredients together in a bowl.

Serve Kofta on the side of the already prepared mix.

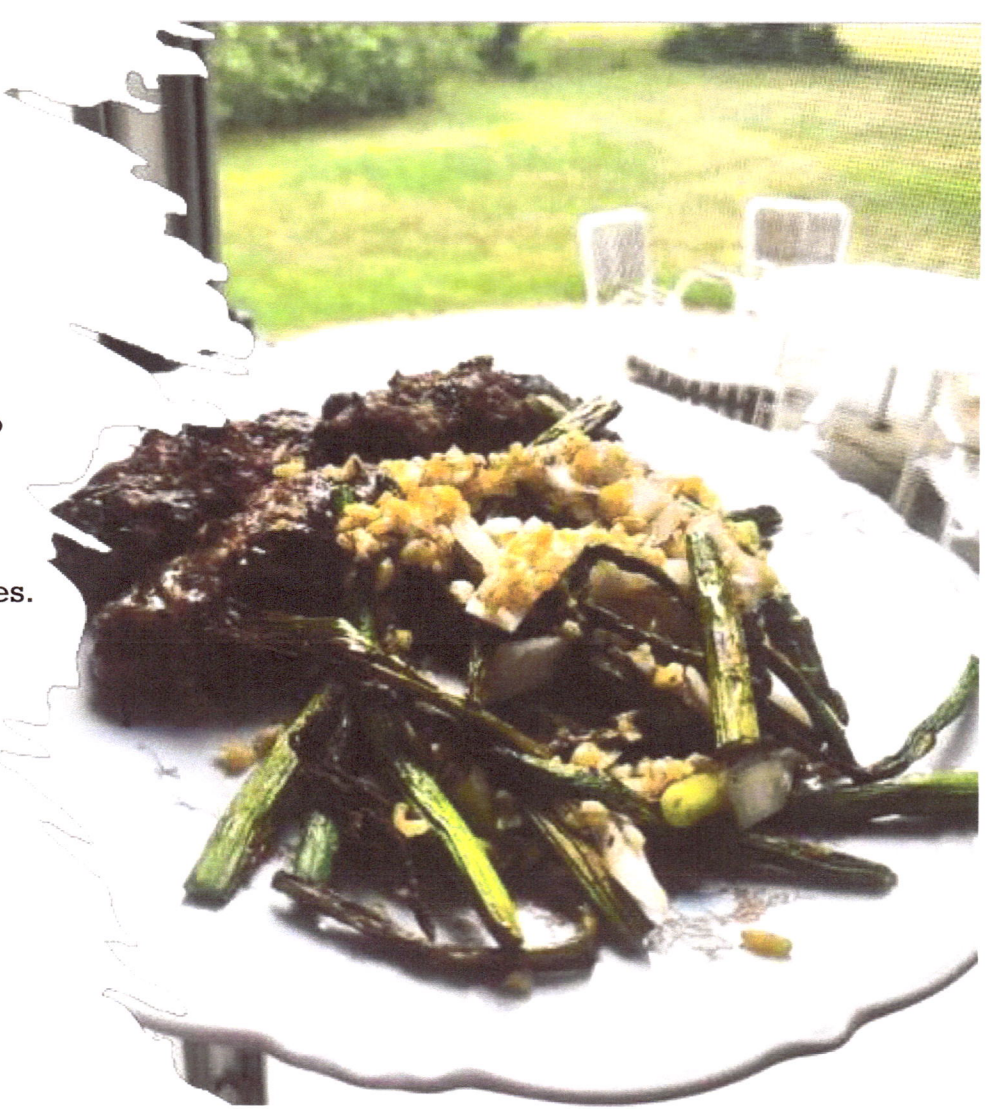

Recipes Mediterranean Inspired

2. KOFTA/ POTATOES. TOMATO PUREE'

Ingredients:
For Kofta: one pound of Ground beef mixed with 1 teaspoon of tomato puree, one diced onion and half a parsley with ¼ TSP of all spice.
Grill Kofta and set aside
2 medium-sized potatoes, half boiled, cut into thick slices, sprinkled with salt and pepper.
2 tomatoes cut into rounds.
2 onions, cut thick in rounds.
1 TSP of hot pepper puree
A mix of tomato puree with salt, pepper, one clove of garlic, 1 TBSP of olive oil.
A drizzle of pomegranate molasses.
Bake for 45 minutes the already half-boiled potatoes, the already cut onions, and tomatoes in a dishpan with 1 TBSP of oil, cover with foil.
Bake all in an oven heated to 350 degrees.
Grill the Kofta after making them in finger shapes for 12 minutes, 6 minutes a side.
Spread on each dis a TBSP of the tomato puree mix.
Place the baked potatoes, onions, and tomatoes on top of the puree, place grilled Kofta fingers.
Drizzle the whole dish with pomegranate molasses.

My understanding of this old existing recipe is that the potatoes are half-boiled and then baked. The Kofta is mixed with hot pepper and tomato puree. The extra twist is that the tomato puree is pasted on the plate under the kofta and potato, not soaked with sauce like the original one.

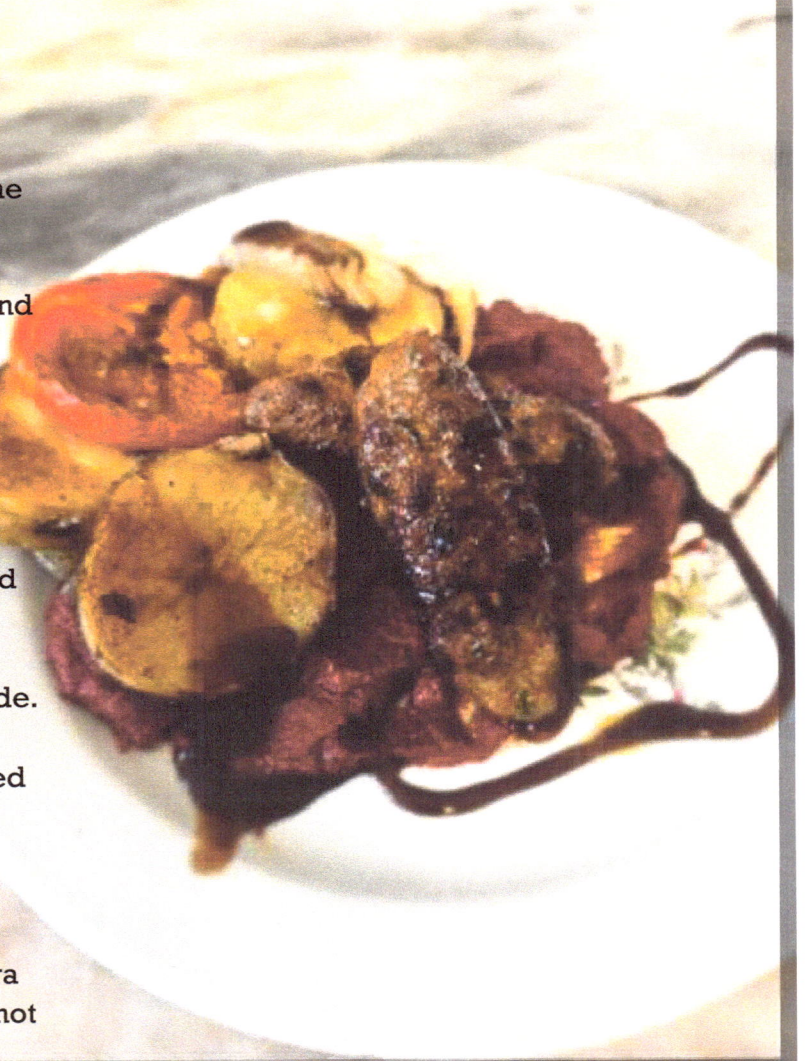

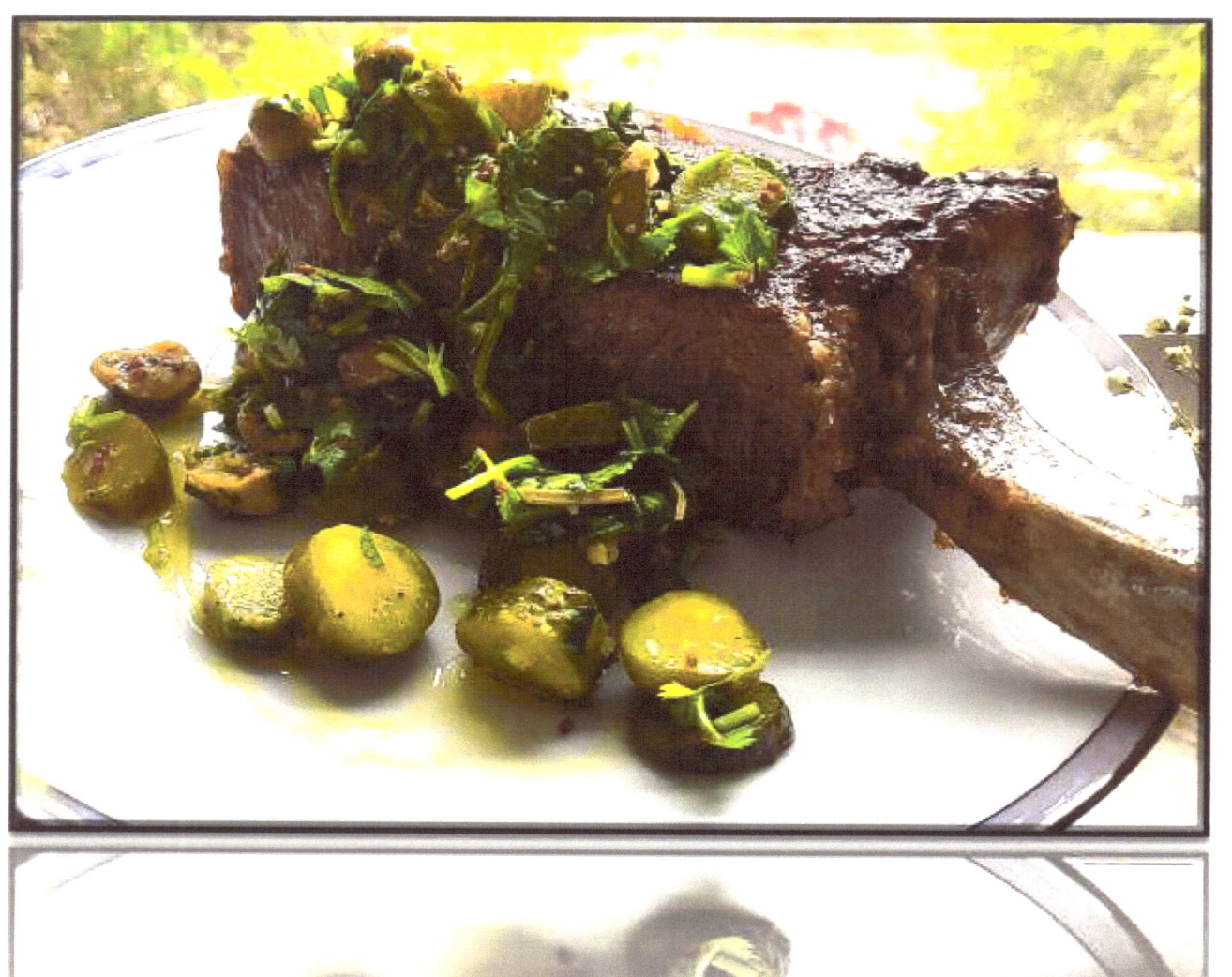

3. STEAK

Ingredients:
One pound and half pounds of bone-in steak. Peppered and salted. Leave it at room temperature for an hour.
Grill on medium heat or to your liking.
3 cucumber pickle fingers cut in rounds
Diced a bunch of cilantro
Juice of one lemon
2 TBSP of olive oil
2 TBSP of diced green olives
 Mix all ingredients together in a bowl.
Place the mix on top of the already grilled steak.
Serve this dish alongside the baked or mashed potatoes.

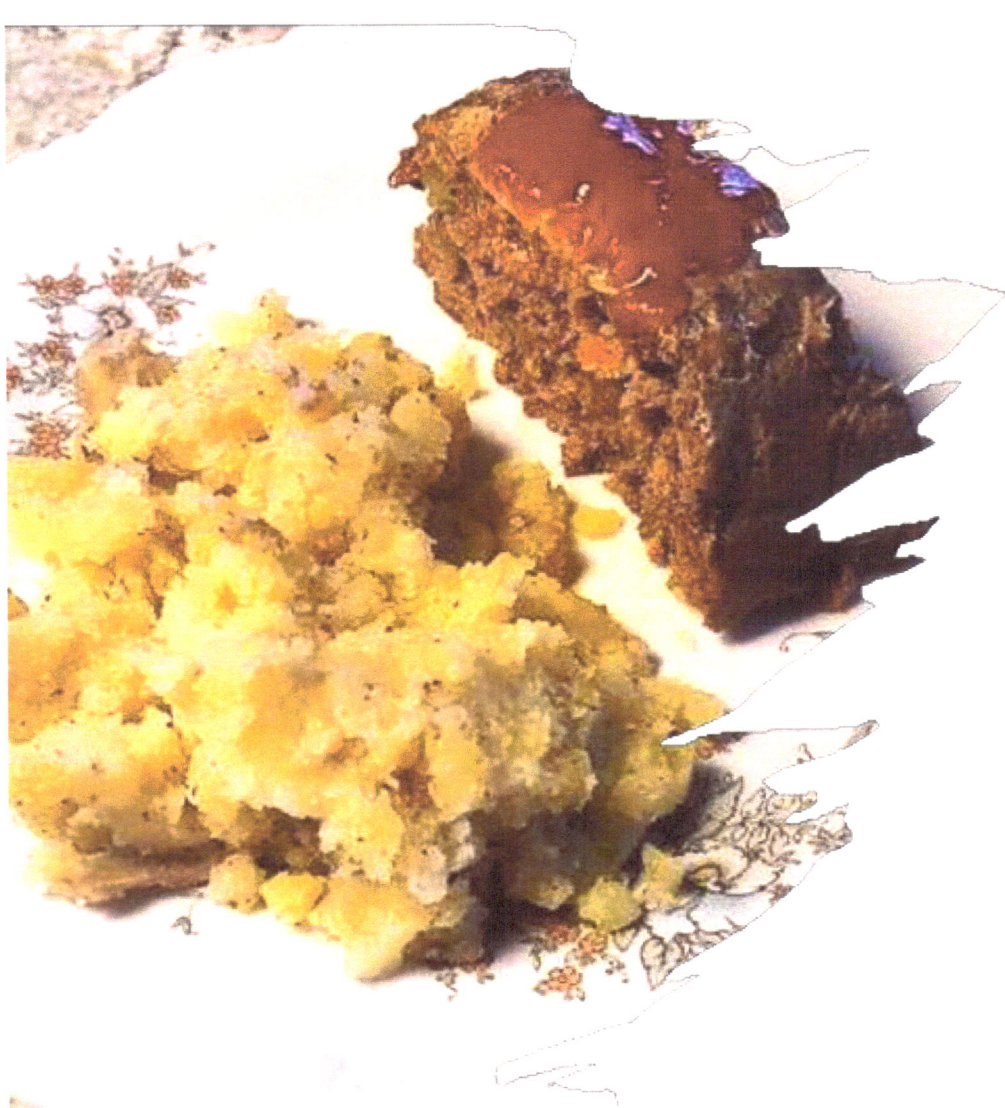

4. MEATLOAF

Ingredients:
1 TBSP of Zaatar
4 cloves of garlic
One pound of ground beef salted, peppered
1 TBSP of diced green olives
1 TBSP of tomato puree.'
1/4 cup of Ketchup
1 onion, diced and sautéed until wilted.
1 TSP of hot pepper puree
Mashed potatoes.

For the meatloaf:

Mix all ingredients together, place the meat mixture into a small pan.

Cover with foil and bake in the oven for an hour. Serve with ketchup on top.

For the mashed potatoes:

Leave the skin on 2 potatoes, boil them for about 45 minutes, or until tender. Once cooked, mash them in the pot, then add 2 cloves of garlic and a generous sliver of butter.

Mix well and serve alongside the meatloaf.

My addition to this old existing recipe is the hot pepper puree and Zaatar, and olives.

5. SOJOK, FREEKEH

Ingredients:

Diced, sauteed Sojok (Lebanese spiced hot dogs).

Boiled and strained one cup of Freekeh.

2 Cucumbers cut into rounds.

Diced 4 stems of green onion.

1 TBSP of white vinegar.

2 TBSP of olive oil.

Mix all ingredients and arrange the cucumber on top.

Bon Appetit

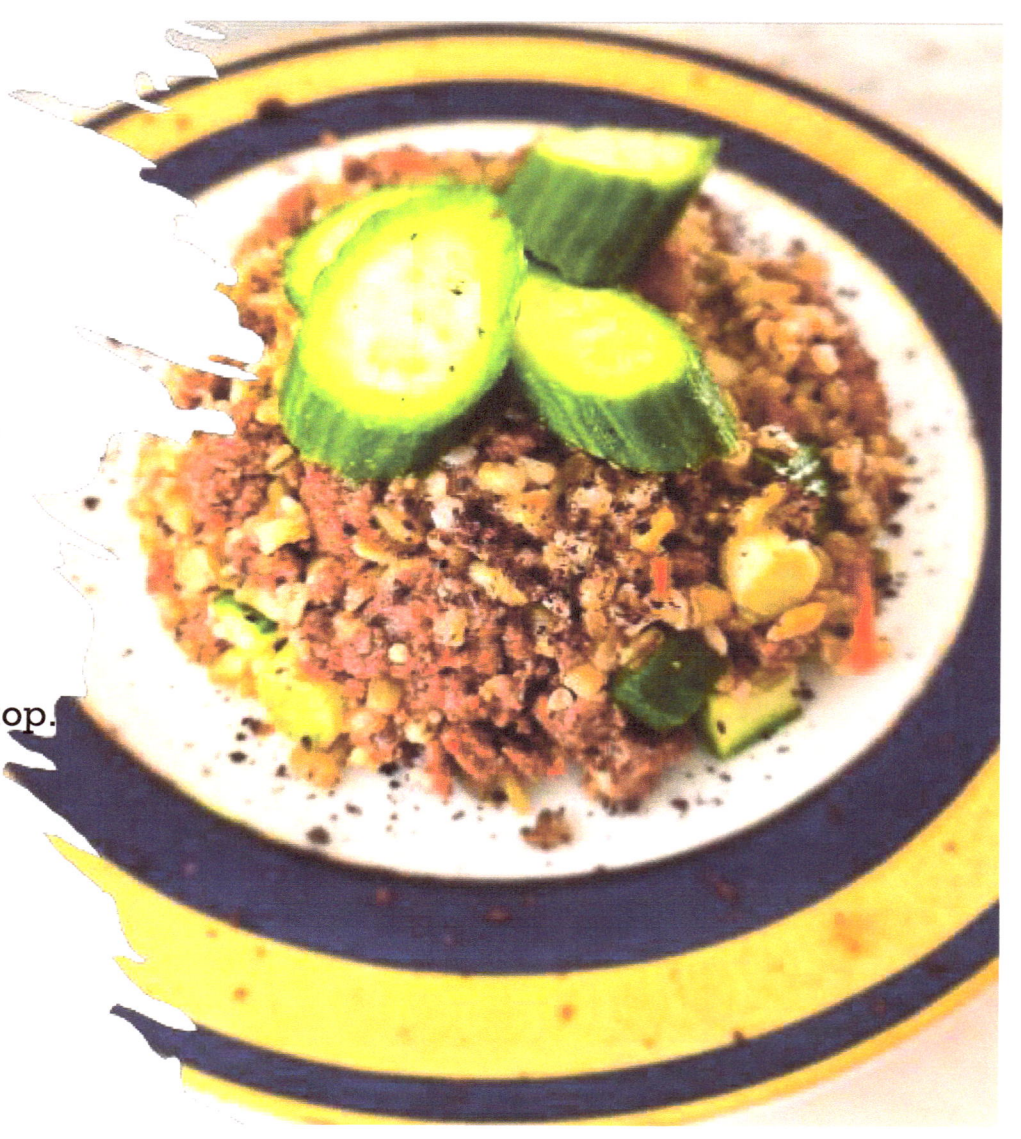

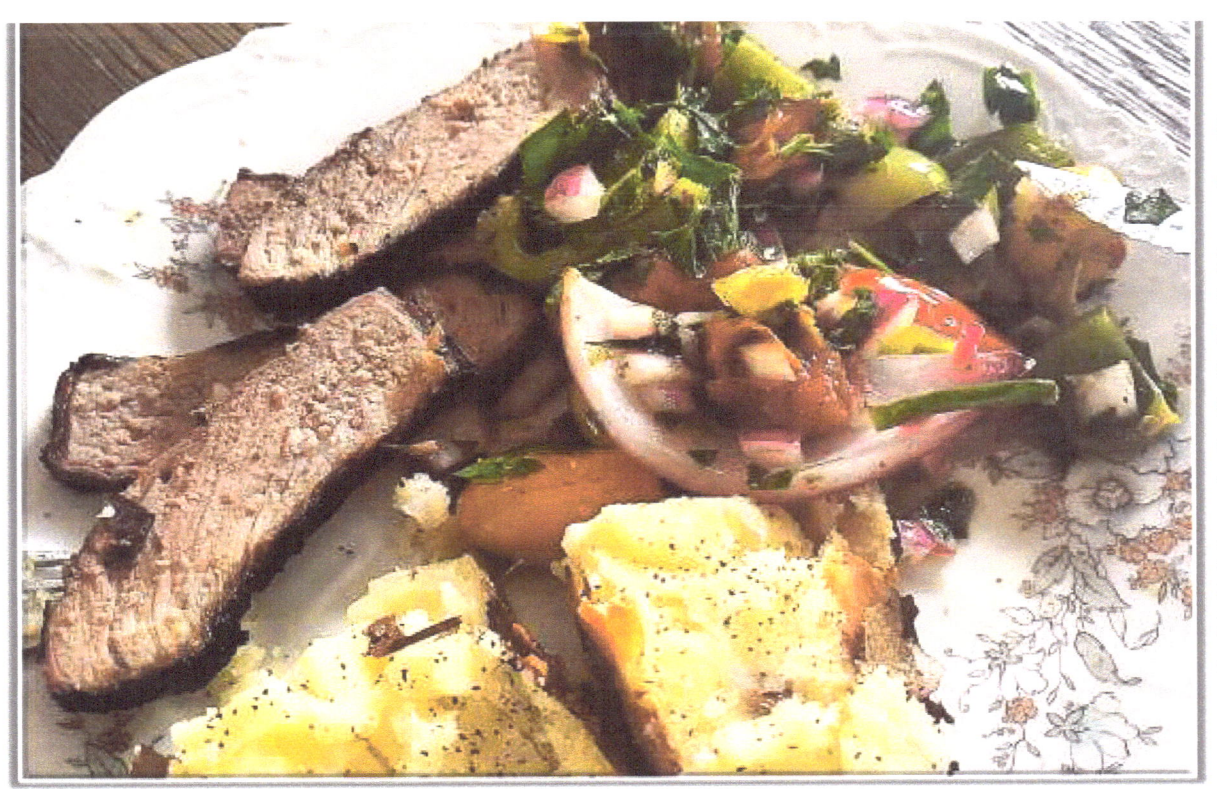

6. STEAK.
ONIONS POTATOES. OLIVES

Ingredients:
Grill one pound of salted, peppered steak on medium heat for 7 minutes a side or to your liking.
Grill 2 heads of medium-sized potatoes for an hour
Cut in rounds a half of a red onion
dice half a bunch of cilantro,
dice half a green pepper
1 TBSP spoon of green olives
Juice of one lemon
3 TBSP of olive oil.
Mix all ingredients in a bowl. Serve on top of already cut steak and grilled potatoes.

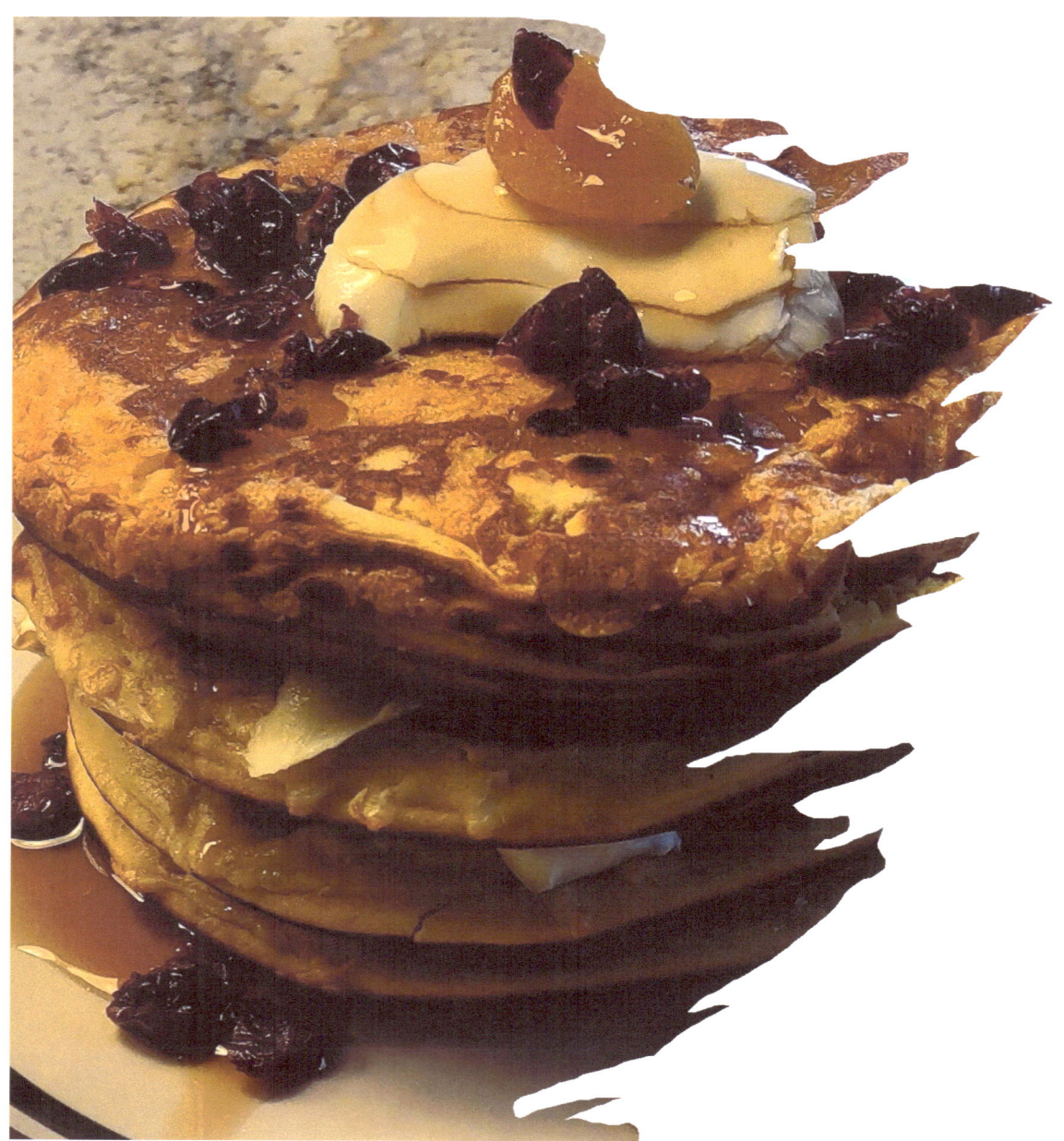

Breakfast

1. PANCAKE, ZAATAR, YOGURT

Ingredients:
Pancake made in a small pan using ***chickpea flour***
One cup per pancake of Plain, nonfat dry yogurt
2 TBSP of Zaatar with olive oil
1 TBSP of pitted green olives
1 TBSP olive oil
Take an already-made pancake and cut in half.
Spread the yogurt on one side along with olives on top.
Spread the mixed zaatar with olive oil on the other side.
Drizzle everything with 1 TBSP olive oil.

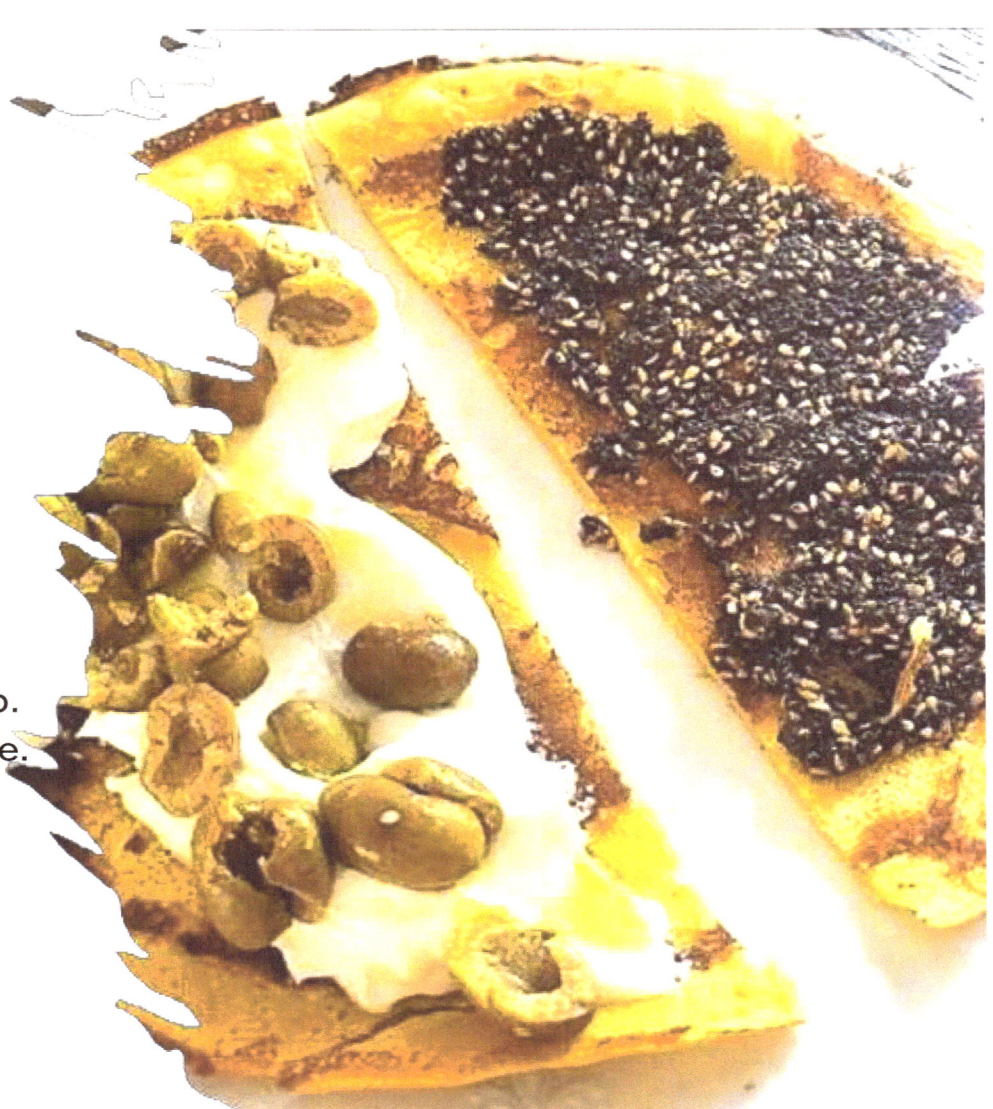

2. ZUCCHINI, CHEESE

Ingredients:

Sliced of mozzarella or Halloumi cheese

4 grilled zucchini, salted, peppered, sliced long, grilled on medium heat

1/4 TBSP paprika

1/4 TBSP of cayenne pepper

Drizzle of pomegranate molasses

3 stems of chopped scallions

Place cheese on top of every slice of already grilled zucchini

Heat for a few minutes until cheese slightly melts.

Sprinkle all with salt & pepper, with the chopped scallions, cayenne, and paprika

Drizzle all with pomegranate molasses.

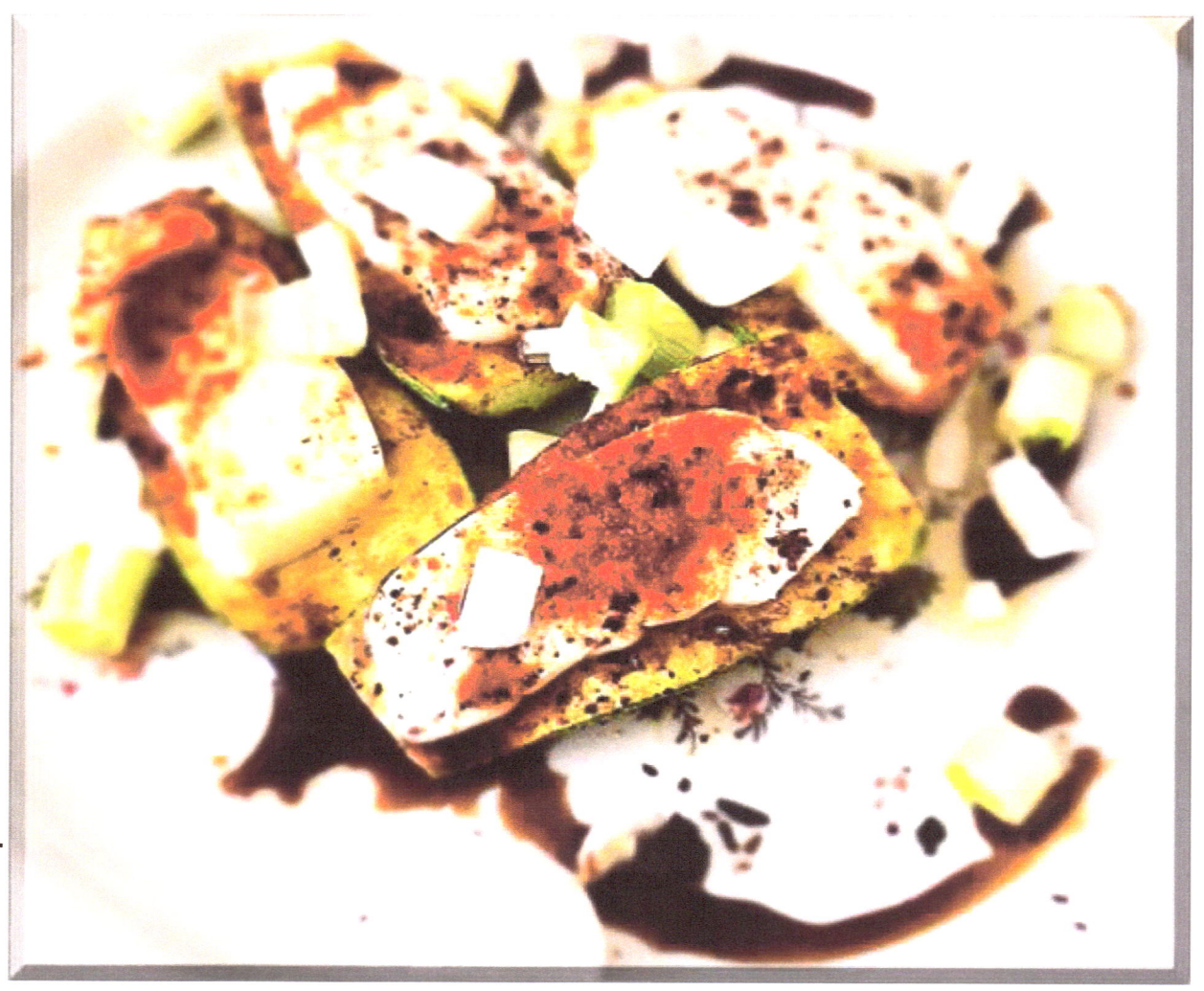

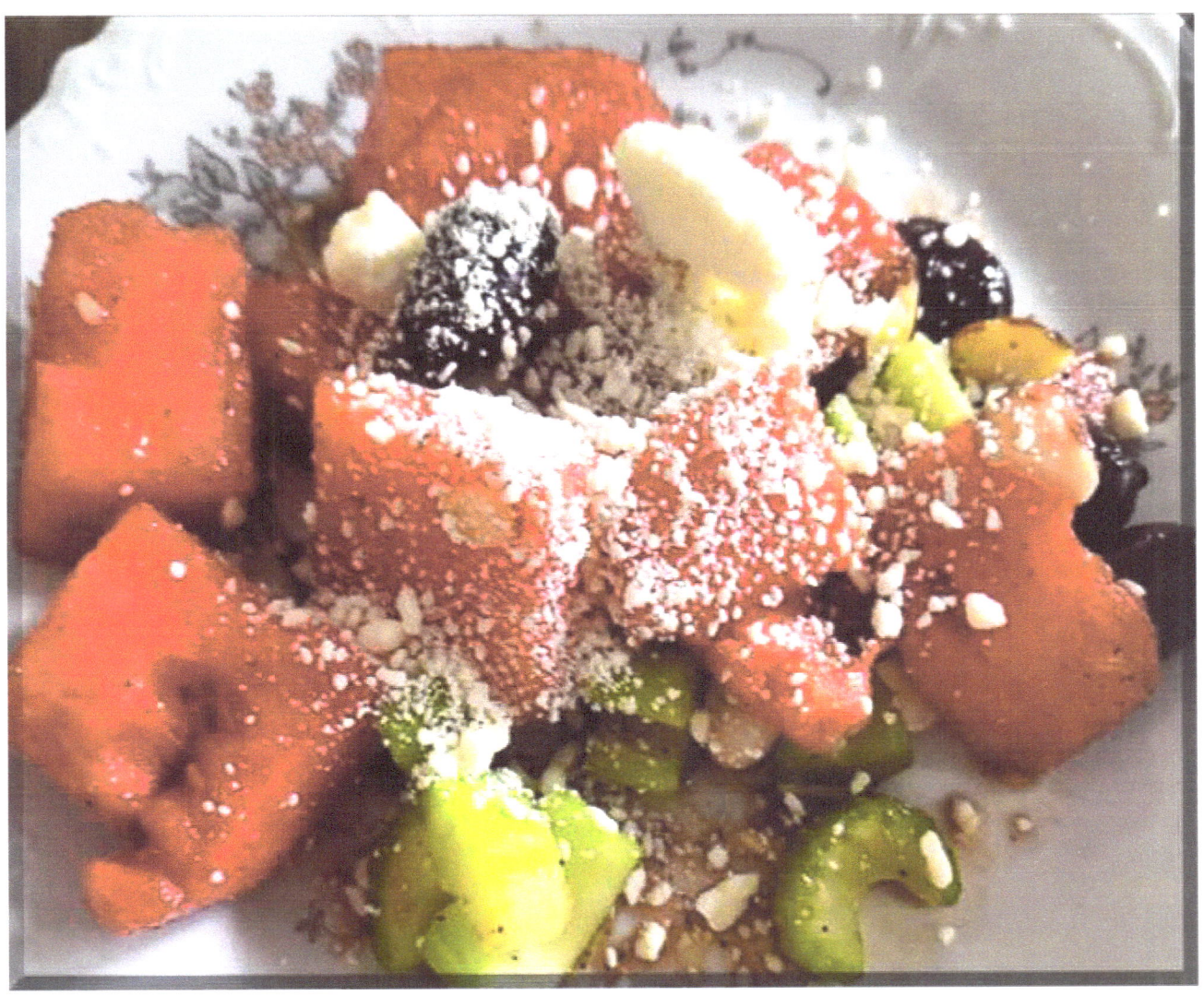

3. WATERMELON. CHEESE

Ingredients:
Watermelon piece for each person
Diced ¾ cup of celery
Diced ½ a cup of black Kalamata olives
½ a cup of crumbled feta cheese
Drizzle of balsamic vinegar and olive oil
Salt and pepper
Mix all ingredients together.
Serve alongside the sliced watermelon.

4. PANCAKE. CHEESE . APRICOTS

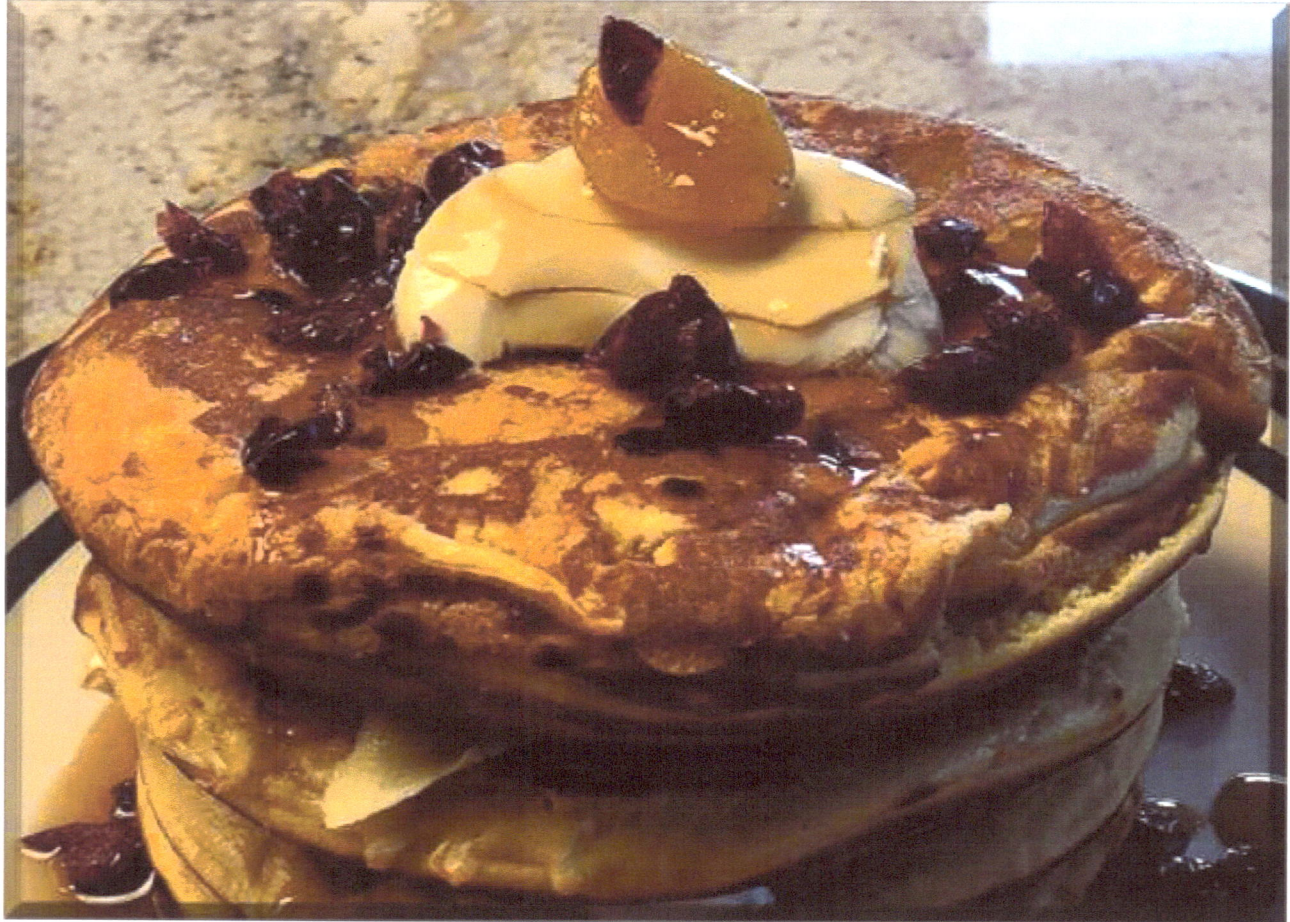

Ingredients:

4 already-made pancakes using **chickpea flour.**

¾ cup of cranberries.

2 slices of Brie cheese, cut into chunks for each pancake layer.

¾ cup of dried apricots. Placed alongside with the cheese between the pancake layers.

¼ cup of maple syrup or honey Stack

Place the brie cheese and apricots between pancake layers, add cranberries on top, drizzle with maple syrup or honey.

Recipes Mediterranean Inspired

5. EGGS, ZAATAR

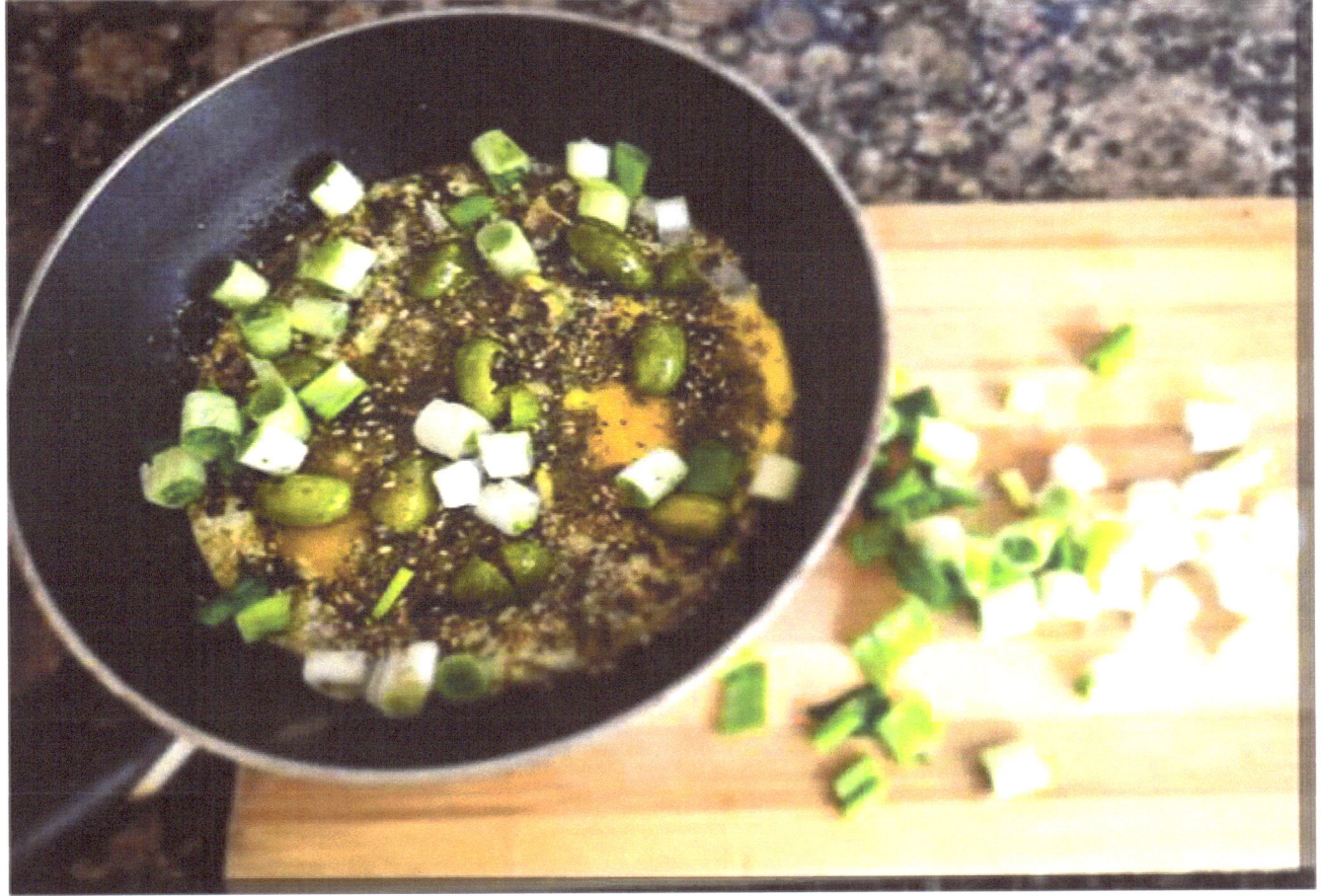

Ingredients:
2 eggs per person, salted, peppered, fried with 1 TBSP of olive oil,
¼ cup of pitted green olives
3 stems of diced green onions
1 TBSP of Zaatar
In the middle of frying the eggs, sprinkle all ingredients on top of the eggs.
Enjoy!!

6. FRENCH TOAST / SAVORY, SWEET

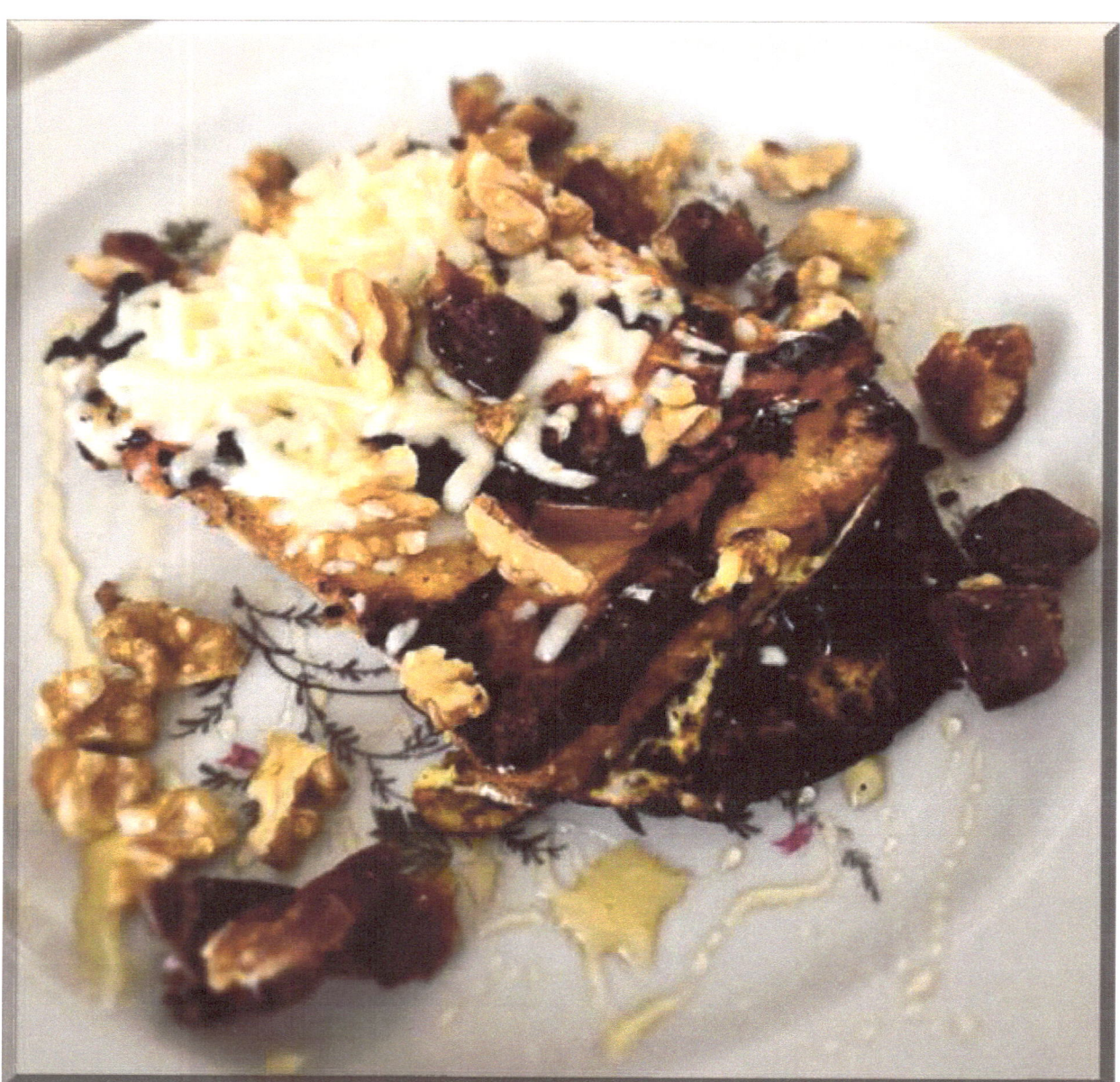

Ingredients:
Brioche toast.
2 eggs beaten with 1 cup of milk.
Pinch of salt and pepper.
1 tomato cut into thick slices.
4 dates pitted, chopped.
One handful of chopped walnuts.
½ a cup of shredded cheese, Mozzarella, or cheddar.
 slivers of butter
1 TBSP of honey
Melt the butter in a heated pan. Add 2 slices of tomato (one for each toast) and cook until they wilt.
Place the dipped toasts in the milk and egg mix over each tomatoes. Cook for 3 minutes.
Flip the toast, cook for an additional 3 minutes
Add cheese on top, cook until slightly melted.
Serve each toast on a plate, sprinkle with chopped dates and walnut, drizzle with honey.

7. YOGURT. LENTILS. PISTACHIOS

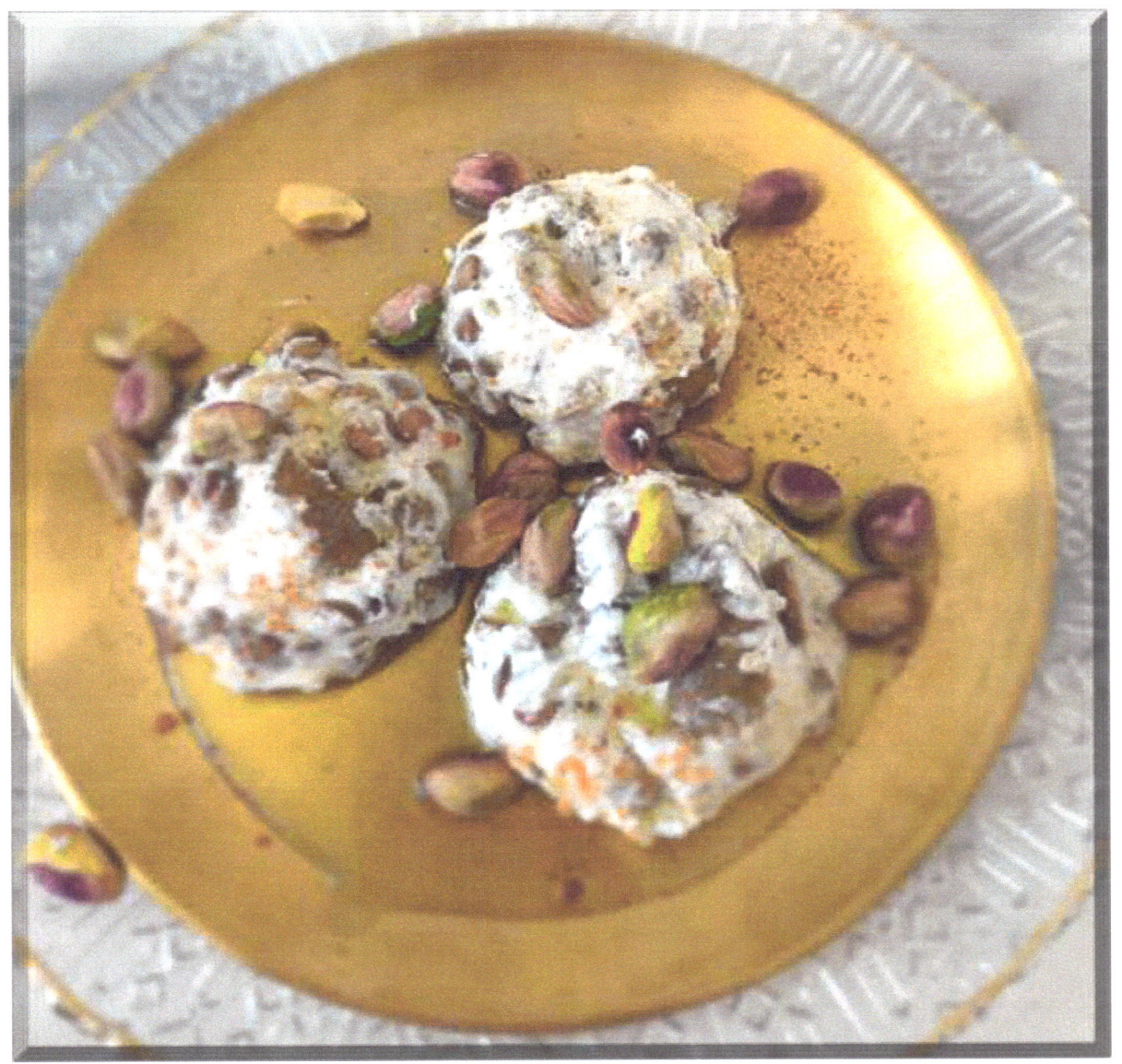

1. 2 TBSP of nonfat Greek yogurt
2. 2 cloves of minced garlic
3. 2 TBSP of extra virgin olive oil
4. ¼ cup of boiled strained lentils
5. Pinch of salt & pepper
6. 1 TBSP of raw pistachios

Mix all ingredients together, use ice cream scoop to create balls to serve. Sprinkle with pistachios

Bon Appetit!

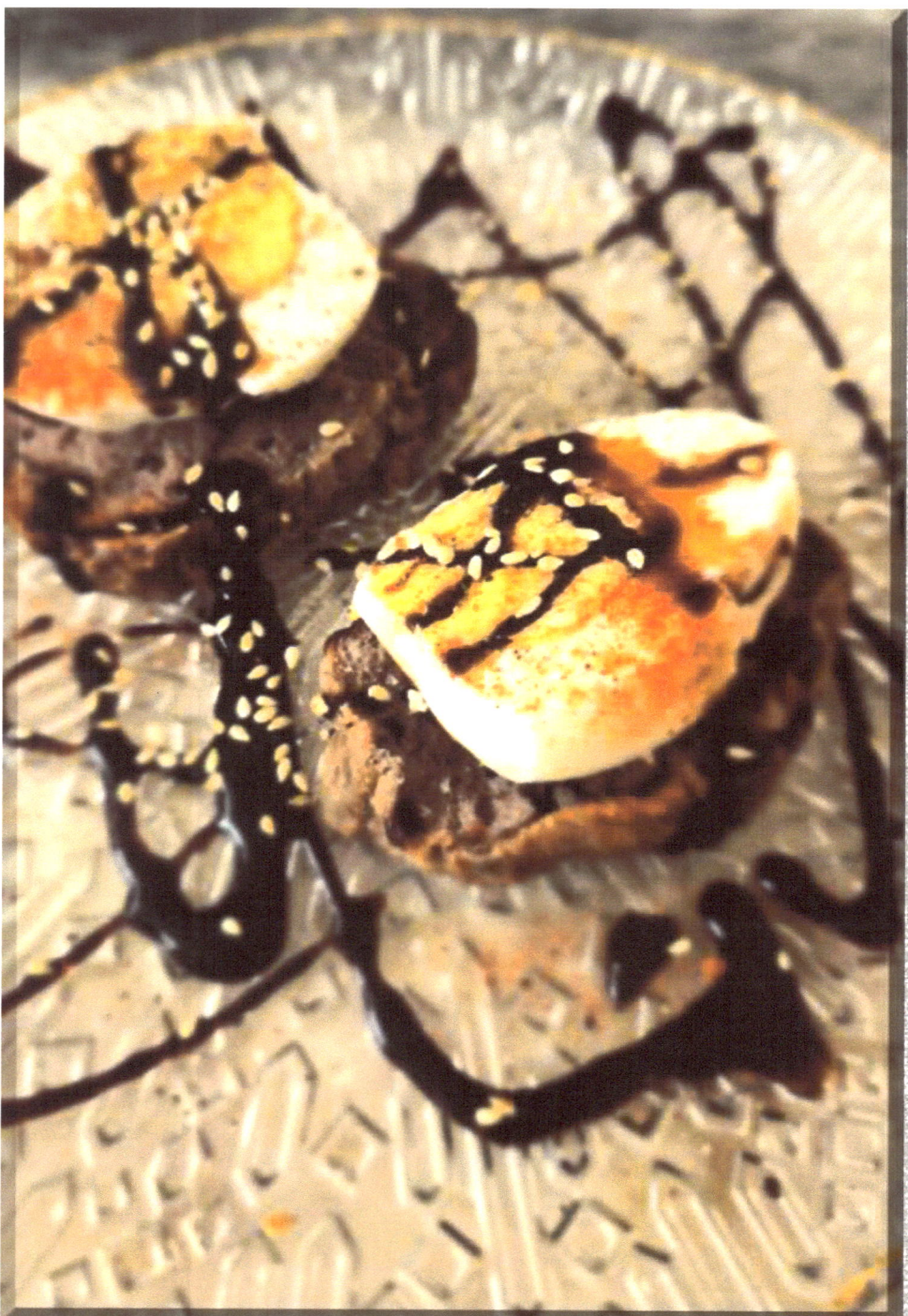

8. Beef. Eggs

Ingredients:

1 boiled egg cut in half

Salt & pepper

¼ TSP of sesame seeds

A drizzle of carob sauce

Ground beef cut in rounds, made with salt & pepper, 4 cloves of minced garlic for every 1 pound.

The beef is formed in a chunky finger shape, sprinkled with flour on all sides then browned on 4 sides in a pan with a drizzle of olive oil then baked in oven on a medium heat for 40 min covered with foil.

Beef is cut in rounds when it's done and cooled.

Place half an egg on every beef slice

Sprinkle with salt & pepper & sesame seeds

Drizzle all dish with carob sauce.

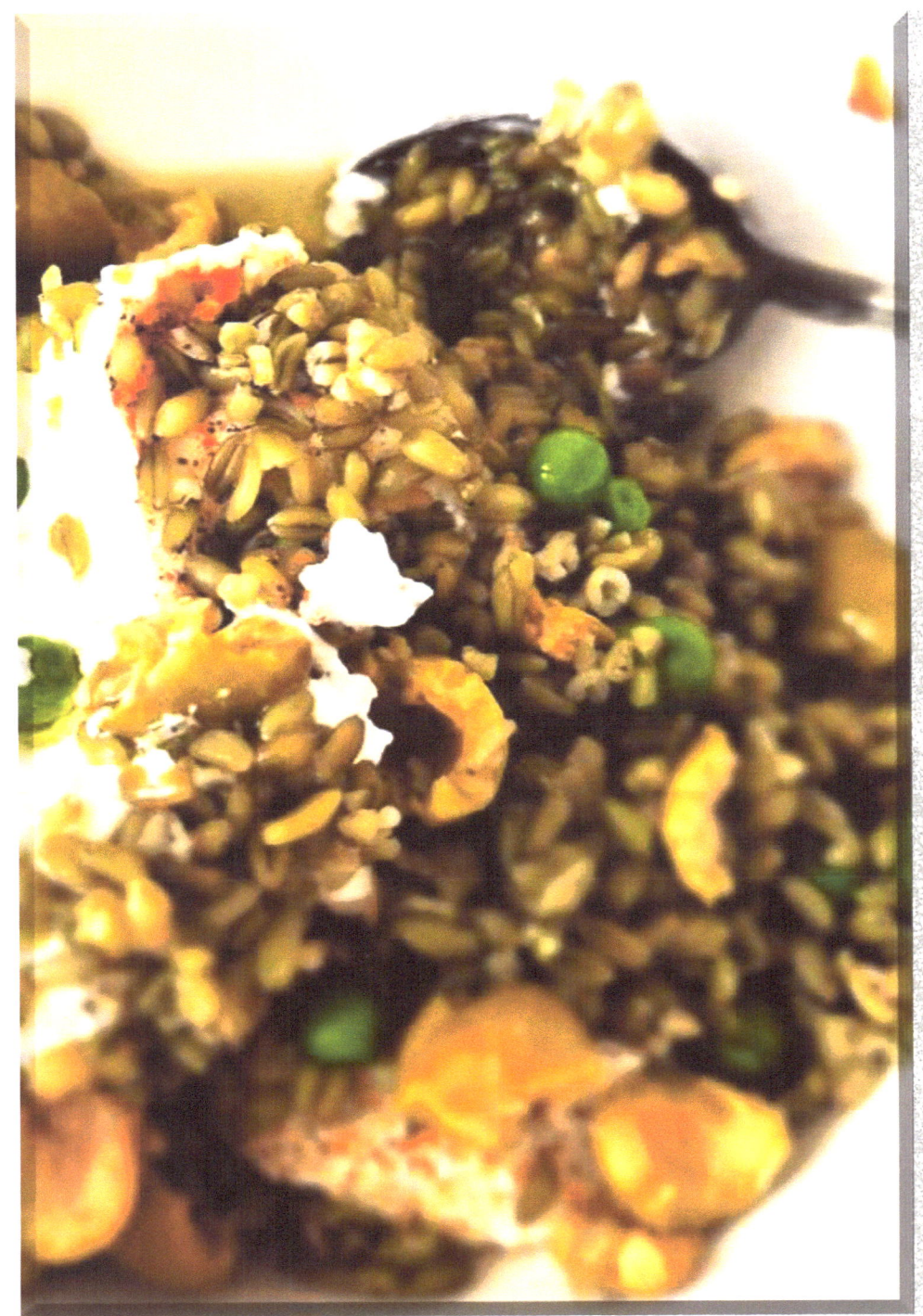

9. Freekeh. Yogurt

Ingredients:

2 TBSP of nonfat Greek yogurt

¼ cup of already boiled & strained Freekeh

2 TBSP of frozen peas thawed

2 TBSP of pitted olives

1 TBSP of olive oil

Salt & pepper

1 Clove of minced garlic

Mix all ingredients together.

Enjoy!

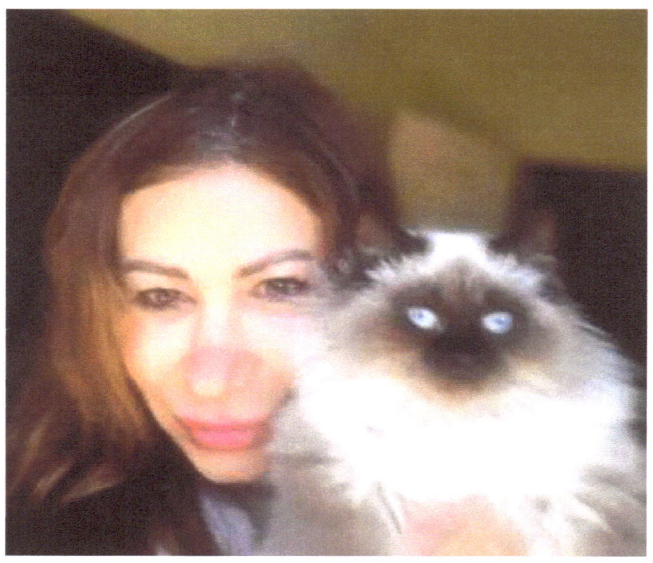

Born in Lebanon on the sea on the northern coastline, the author enjoyed growing up a variety of local dishes made first by her mom, and second by local restaurants.
Meals, made with fresh produce, freshly cut red meat, freshly slaughtered chickens, and freshly caught seafood.
Meals made using lots of Mediterranean ingredients like legumes (beans/ grains), olive oil, lemon juice, garlic, and onions.
As time passed by, she realized that these ingredients were missing from most of the recipes she tasted in different countries! Basic ingredients that are not only healthy to have but also elevate the dish from basic plain flavor to something truly flavorful!
Here we go, have some of my recipes and enjoy!!

Lina Khatib
Interior Architect/ Health Conscience